# Great Ormond Street [ of Paediatric Vasc Anomalies

This new text from the Great Street Hospital team is a practical guide to the current multidisciplinary clinical management of paediatric vascular anomalies. Aiming to share their valuable expertise, this book offers a much-needed clinical resource for the multidisciplinary team. From haematology to orbital vascular malformations, this text presents a comprehensive overview of paediatric vascular anomalies, offering a wealth of tips from practical experience. Including illustrations from current practice, this book is a valuable addition to all those involved in the care of children with these rare conditions.

**Neil W. Bulstrode BSc (Hons) MBBS MD FRCS (Plast)**, Consultant Plastic Surgeon, Great Ormond Street Hospital for Children; Honorary Associate Professor, UCL GOS Institute of Child Health, London, UK

**Alex Barnacle MB FRCR**, Consultant Paediatric Interventional Radiologist, Great Ormond Street Hospital for Children, London, UK

**Maanasa Polubothu BSc MBChB MSc PhD FRCPCH**, Consultant in Paediatric Dermatology, Great Ormond Street Hospital for Children; Honorary Associate Professor, Genetics & Genomic Medicine, UCL GOS Institute of Child Health, London, UK

# Great Ormond Street Handbook Series

**Great Ormond Street Handbook of Paediatrics, Second Edition**
*Edited by Stephan Strobel, Lewis Spitz, and Stephen D. Marks*

**Great Ormond Street Handbook of Congenital Ear Deformities**
An Illustrated Surgical Guide
*Neil W. Bulstrode and Ahmed Salah Mazeed*

**Great Ormond Street Handbook of Paediatric Vascular Anomalies: An Illustrated Guide to Clinical Management**
*Edited by Neil W. Bulstrode, Alex Barnacle, and Maanasa Polubothu*

For more information about this series, please visit: https://www.routledge.com/Great-Ormond-Street-Handbook-Series/book-series/GOSH

# Great Ormond Street Handbook of Paediatric Vascular Anomalies

## An Illustrated Guide to Clinical Management

Edited by

**Neil W. Bulstrode**

**Alex Barnacle**

**Maanasa Polubothu**

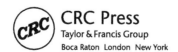

CRC Press
Taylor & Francis Group
Boca Raton London New York

CRC Press is an imprint of the
Taylor & Francis Group, an **informa** business

Cover image: Shutterstock Image ID 2212503203

First edition published 2024

by CRC Press
6000 Broken Sound Parkway NW, Suite 300, Boca Raton, FL 33487-2742

and by CRC Press
4 Park Square, Milton Park, Abingdon, Oxon, OX14 4RN
*CRC Press is an imprint of Taylor & Francis Group, LLC*

Library of Congress Cataloging-in-Publication Data

Names: Bulstrode, Neil, editor. | Barnacle, Alex, editor. | Polubothu, Maanasa, editor. | Great Ormond Street Hospital for Children (London, England), issuing body.
Title: Great Ormond Street handbook of paediatric vascular anomalies : an illustrated guide to clinical management / edited by Neil Bulstrode, Alex Barnacle, and Maanasa Polubothu.
Other titles: Handbook of paediatric vascular anomalies
Description: First edition. | Boca Raton : CRC Press, 2023. | Includes bibliographical references and index. | Summary: "This new text from the Great Ormond Street Hospital team is a practical guide to the current multi-disciplinary clinical management of paediatric vascular anomalies. Aiming to share their valuable expertise, this book offers a much-needed clinical resource for the multi-disciplinary team. From haematology to orbital vascular malformations, this text provides a comprehensive overview of paediatric vascular anomalies, offering a wealth of tips from practical experience. Including illustrations from current practice, this book is a valuable addition to all those involved in the care of children with these rare conditions"-- Provided by publisher.
Identifiers: LCCN 2023013461 (print) | LCCN 2023013462 (ebook) | ISBN 9781032190297 (hardback) | ISBN 9781032190280 (paperback) | ISBN 9781003257417 (ebook)
Subjects: MESH: Vascular Malformations--therapy | Vascular Malformations--diagnosis | Child | Infant | Handbook
Classification: LCC RJ496.C45 (print) | LCC RJ496.C45 (ebook) | NLM WG 39 | DDC 618.9/281--dc23/eng/20230404
LC record available at https://lccn.loc.gov/2023013461
LC ebook record available at https://lccn.loc.gov/2023013462

ISBN: 978-1-032-19029-7 (hbk)
ISBN: 978-1-032-19028-0 (pbk)
ISBN: 978-1-003-25741-7 (ebk)

DOI: 10.1201/9781003257417

Typeset in ITC Galliard
by Deanta Global Publishing Services, Chennai, India

# Contents

Contents

# Foreword

In the mid-1970s, a young Anglo-American team stumbled onto the nascent field of vascular anomalies. I was studying cellular turnover in vascular lesions in Judah Folkman's laboratory. Tony Young had written his thesis on combined vascular 'birthmarks' in the limbs and came to Boston as a visiting fellow from St. Thomas. Tony and I immediately expressed a mutual fascination with vascular anomalies. We agreed the subject was a terminological chamber of horrors – every blue, pink, or red vascular lesion was called 'hemangioma'. We organized biennial Vascular Anomaly Workshop meetings that grew to become the International Society for the Study of Vascular Anomalies (ISSVA). The organization is thriving beyond our imagination – it even has its own journal called *JOVA*.

At the 11th ISSVA meeting in Rome (1996), the biological classification of vascular anomalies as 'tumors' and 'malformations' was accepted. This binary scheme cleared the clouds of nosological confusion; now we could speak with a common tongue. Vascular anomalies centers emerged worldwide in major university children's (and some adult) hospitals. Medical and surgical specialists gathered in interdisciplinary teams to deliberate how to care for these patients.

Given infantile hemangioma's remarkable cellular proliferation and programmed cell death, I presumed the etiology of this most common pediatric tumor would be easily solved. Hemangioma endothelium exhibits distinctive immunostaining for the glucose transporter (GLUT-1). The marker is absent in 'congenital hemangiomas' – tumors that arise *in utero* and either involute rapidly (RICH) or persist (NICH). Another pathogenic clue is accelerated regression when infantile hemangioma is treated early with a corticosteroid or a beta-blocker. There are also hints in the uncommon association of hemangioma with malformative anomalies: PHACES in the head/neck and LUMBAR in the ventral-caudal region. The causal hypothesis is a somatic mutation in a hemangioma stem cell – which can differentiate into endothelial cells, pericytes, and adipocytes – but the trigger for 'hemangiogenesis' remains unknown.

In contrast, the revolution in molecular genetics exploded our understanding of vascular malformations. Families with inherited vascular lesions clustered in centers and, thus, enabled gene hunting. The genetic mutations (both germline and somatic) responsible for most vascular malformations have been tracked down. Standard vascular anomaly gene panels are available for identifying mutations utilizing blood, fresh tissue, or formalin-fixed specimens. But genetic-phenotypic correlations are often not straightforward. For example, somatic *PIK3CA* mutations are common in isolated lymphatic malformations as well as in complex vascular disorders with an LM component, such as Klippel–Trenaunay syndrome, CLOVES, and FAVA. Mutations in *PIK3CA* (and *TIE2*) are also found in sporadic venous malformations. *GNAQ* activating mutations cause capillary malformations (and Sturge–Weber syndrome) but are also detected in NICH, RICH, and pyogenic granuloma. RASopathies are caused by somatic mutations in the RAS/MAPK pathway, resulting in vascular anomalies with overlapping features such as *NRAS* in KLA, *RASA1* in CCM-AVM, and *KRAS* in AVM. Mutations in *MAP2K1*, *KRAS*, and *BRAF* are also found in AVMs, while *KRAS*, *NRAS*, and *BRAF* are responsible for pyogenic granuloma.

Understanding mutations that give rise to vascular malformations (most are gain-of-function) and their downstream effects ushered in a new era of pharmacological therapy. Many of the drugs were already used by oncologists. Medical therapy may not 'cure' a vascular anomaly. The goal is to 'control' expansion, bleeding, infection, overgrowth, and recurrence. Targeted pharmacological treatment has begun to diminish the role of traditional interventional radiology procedures such as embolization and sclerotherapy. Drugs can also help surgeons – and sometimes put them 'out of business'.

A colleague cannot be cajoled or assigned to a vascular anomalies team. The field attracts physicians with a genetic predisposition to care for these challenging and mysterious afflictions.

**John B. Mulliken MD, FACS, Hon FRCS (Engl)**
Boston Children's Hospital
Harvard Medical School

# Preface

The management of vascular anomalies is a team event, and the *Great Ormond Street Handbook of Paediatric Vascular Anomalies* has been born out of the experience of our incredible team of dermatologists, radiologists, physicians, surgeons, nurses, therapists, psychologists, and others. Of course, our patients and their parents and families are at the centre, always inspiring us to do better. The Great Ormond Street team evolved from two giants of paediatric dermatology, Dr David Atherton and the late Professor John Harper, growing into this centre of excellence treating children with the most complex of vascular anomalies and contributing to the development of pioneering multidisciplinary treatments and research in this field. This approach has included many international collaborations, with numerous doctors who trained with us returning to their local units in the UK and abroad and using this template to build their own specialist units. Our team is, in turn, immensely grateful for the training, wisdom, and expertise that vascular anomalies experts across the globe have shared with us over the years, answering our questions with endless patience, and helping us to grow and learn.

The management of vascular anomalies has changed dramatically over the past 50 years, with several key milestones in that time. These include Professor John Mulliken's revolutionary classification of these diseases, which both improved our understanding of this field and enabled us to agree on nomenclature, thereby facilitating more accurate discussions between teams and safer care for patients. The serendipitous discovery that beta-blockers could reverse the growth phase of infantile haemangiomas was, according to John Harper, 'the most important advance in paediatric dermatology in his clinical lifetime'. Also in those 50 years, interventional radiology was born as a specialty, opening up innovative and novel ways of imaging and treating many of these conditions. Over the past 10 years, advances in molecular genetics have enabled the discovery of the genetic basis of many vascular anomalies, accelerating our understanding of the underlying pathogenesis and enabling the development of a personalised medicine approach, with the successful use of targeted medical therapies now possible in some cohorts. There are many more developments, of course, that will be highlighted in this book, including the constant drive to make small improvements in the patient's journey.

The editors and authors of this book wanted to convey our centre's ethos of bringing all the team members' knowledge to bear on the individual patient and their condition. We want to thank all the members of the team who all play key roles. The open discussions that occur in our multidisciplinary meetings honestly debate the treatment options available, keep the child at the centre of our focus, and create a rich forum for innovation and research to thrive. Respect for the specialist skills brought to the table allows everyone to give their opinion knowing they will be supported and backed by the team. In this complex field of medicine, it is rare for one centre to have all the answers, and as children grow, both their condition and their personal needs change.

Our aim is that this book will inspire more clinical teams to care for children with complex vascular anomalies and give them confidence in their approach to the conditions discussed. We hope that teams will see that sharing the burden between specialties will improve both clinical outcomes and the patient's experience.

*Neil W. Bulstrode*
*Alex Barnacle*
*Maanasa Polubothu*

# Contributors

**Alex Barnacle** MB FRCR
Consultant Paediatric Interventional Radiologist
Great Ormond Street Hospital for Children
London, UK

**Sanjay Bhate** MD MRCP MRCPCH
Consultant Paediatric Neurologist and Lead
    Clinician Neurovascular Service
Great Ormond Street Hospital for Children
and
Honorary Associate Professor in
    Neurosciences
University College London Great Ormond Street
    Institute of Child Health
London, UK

**Neil W. Bulstrode** BSc (Hons) MBBS MD
    FRCS (Plast)
Consultant Plastic Surgeon
Great Ormond Street Hospital for Children
and
Honorary Associate Professor
UCL GOS Institute of Child Health
London, UK

**Sunit Davda** BSc MBBS MRCP FRCR FRCPC
Consultant Interventional Radiologist
Great Ormond Street Hospital for Children
London, UK

**Deborah Eastwood** MB FRCS
Consultant Paediatric Orthopaedic Surgeon
Great Ormond Street Hospital
and
Royal National Orthopaedic Hospital
and
Associate Professor
University College London
London, UK

**Sofia Eriksson** MBChB MRCS
Plastic Surgery Registrar
Great Ormond Street Hospital for Children
London, UK

**Mary Glover** MA FRCP FRCPCH
Consultant Paediatric Dermatologist
Great Ormond Street Hospital for Children
London, UK

**Sri Gore** BSc FRCOphth PGDip Ed
Consultant Ophthalmologist and Oculoplastic
    Surgeon
Great Ormond Street Hospital
and
Honorary Consultant
Moorfields Eye Hospital
London, UK

**Richard J. Hewitt** FRCS (ORL-HNS)
Consultant Paediatric Ear, Nose, and
    Throat; Head and Neck; and Tracheal
    Surgeon
Great Ormond Street Hospital for Children
London, UK

**Greg James** PhD FRCS (Neuro Surg)
Consultant Neurosurgeon and Associate
    Professor
Department of Neurosurgery
Great Ormond Street Hospital
and
Department of Neuroscience, Physiology and
    Pharmacology
University College London
London, UK

**Matthew Lloyd Jones** MBChB FRACS
Consultant Paediatric Plastic Surgeon
Perth Children's Hospital
Perth, Australia

**Mary Mathias** MA MBBS MRCP
    FRCPath MD
Consultant Haematologist
Great Ormond Street Hospital for Children
London, UK

**Kishore Minhas** MBChB MSc FRCR
Consultant Interventional Radiologist
Great Ormond Street Hospital for Children
London, UK

**Claire O'Neill** MD FRCPCH
Specialist Doctor in Paediatric Dermatology
Great Ormond Street Hospital for Children
London, UK

**Jadesola Oyedepo-Babawarun** MBBS FWACP
  (Paeds) MRCPCH
Clinical Fellow
Paediatric Dermatology
Great Ormond Street Hospital for Children
London, UK

**Premal Patel** BSc (Hons) MBBS FRCR
Consultant Interventional Radiologist
Great Ormond Street Hospital for Children
London, UK

**Maanasa Polubothu** BSc MBChB MSc PhD
  FRCPCH
Consultant in Paediatric Dermatology
Great Ormond Street Hospital for Children
and
Honorary Associate Professor
Genetics & Genomic Medicine
UCL GOS Institute of Child Health
London, UK

**Francisco Regel** VBDS MBBS
Senior House Officer
Plastic Surgery
Great Ormond Street Hospital for Children
London, UK

**Adam Rennie** MB BS BMSc FRCR
Consultant Interventional Neuroradiologist
Great Ormond Street Hospital for Children
and
National Hospital for Neurology &
  Neurosurgery, Queen Square
London, UK

**Fergus Robertson** MD MRCP FRCR
Consultant Interventional Neuroradiologist
Great Ormond Street Hospital for Children
and
National Hospital for Neurology &
  Neurosurgery, Queen Square
London, UK

**Amir Sadri** BSc MBChB FRCS
Consultant Plastic Surgeon
Great Ormond Street Hospital for Children
London, UK

**Neil J. Sebire** BBS BClinSci MD FFCI FRCOG
  FRCPath
Professor of Pathology
Great Ormond Street Hospital
Institute of Child Health
University College London
and
Chief Research Information Officer
National Institute of Health and Care
Biomedical Research Centre
London, UK

**Bran Sivakumar** MD (Res) FRCS (Plast)
Consultant Plastic Surgeon
Great Ormond Street Hospital for Children
London, UK

**Lea Solman** MD FRCPCH
Consultant Paediatric Dermatologist
Great Ormond Street Hospital for Children
London, UK

**Kristina Soon** PhD MPsych (Clin) BA (Hons)
  CPsychol
Clinical Psychologist
Great Ormond Street Hospital for Children
and
Associate Teaching Professor
Clinical, Educational and Health Psychology
University College London
London, UK

# 1 Introduction and Classification

Sofia Eriksson, Neil Bulstrode, Neil Sebire, Francisco Regel, Alex Barnacle, Maanasa Polubothu, and Jadesola Oyedepo

## INTRODUCTION

Vascular anomalies cover a wide spectrum of lesions from simple 'birthmarks' to large life-threatening or disfiguring tumours. They are structural abnormalities of the vascular system that occur during vasculogenesis, angiogenesis, and lymphangiogenesis (1). Vascular anomalies often present diagnostic challenges due to their vast phenotypic variability, historically inconsistent nomenclature, and ever-changing classification systems. Misdiagnosis is common (2), and incorrect identification of vascular anomalies is associated with the risk of suboptimal management, as the course of disease and treatment options differ greatly depending on the particular vascular anomaly. Agreeing on a universally accepted classification system and nomenclature has been important to ensure consistent terminology, enabling communications between clinicians and guiding proper management of these patients.

## HISTORY

The majority of vascular anomalies present clinically either at birth or shortly afterward and, hence, have long been termed 'birthmarks'. Descriptive classifications of these 'birthmarks' can be found in ancient folklore which evolved from the belief that a mother's emotions could mark her unborn fetus (3). It was thought that if a mother experienced heightened emotions during pregnancy, the shock might be felt by the fetus and register as a skin blemish, with the mark resembling the object or circumstance which triggered the mother's emotional state. Others believed the mother was to blame for eating too much of certain foods or failing to satisfy certain cravings of food items that looked like the birthmark such as strawberries, raspberries, or cherries. The marks came to be called mother's marks, or *naevus maternus*, and many European languages share this type of term. The French call a birthmark *envie*, a desire; the Italians, *voglia*, a wish or craving. In German, the word is *muttermal*, mother's mark, and in Spanish, *estigma* (3). Terminology based on similarity to foodstuffs continues to exist to the present day with examples such as strawberry haemangioma, port-wine stain, and salmon patch.

More scientific approaches to understanding vascular anomalies started to emerge in the eighteenth century. The earliest pathologic classification was described by Virchow in 1863. He termed all vascular anomalies 'angiomas' and classified them according to their histological architecture into angioma simplex (composed of increased capillaries), angioma cavernosum (the replacement of normal vasculature with large channels), or angioma racemosum (composed of dilated and interconnected vessels) (4). As new vascular pathologies were discovered, terms such as 'haemangioma', 'hamartoma', and 'endothelioma' were created, complicating classification (3).

In a landmark publication on vascular anomalies in 1982, Mulliken and Glowacki proposed separating vascular anomalies into two major classification types based on their pathological characteristics: 'haemangiomas', which were characterised by endothelial proliferation and hyperplasia, and 'malformations', which showed vessel dysplasia but with apparently normal endothelial turnover (5). Despite many other classifications having been proposed since then (Figure 1.1), this model has laid the basis for the

DOI: 10.1201/9781003257417-1

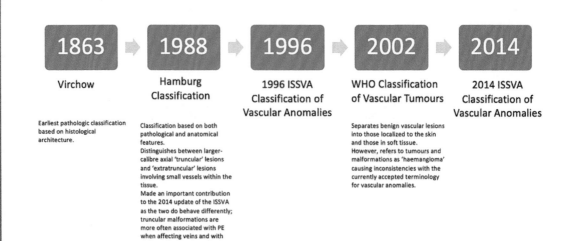

FIGURE 1.1 From Virchov 1863 (4), Hamburg Classification 1988 (6), ISSVA 1996/2014/2018 (7), WHO 2002 (9, 10).

current International Society for the Study of Vascular Anomalies (ISSVA) classification system used today.

The ISSVA classification and the World Health Organization (WHO) classification are the two classification systems most commonly used internationally.

## ISSVA CLASSIFICATION

The ISSVA is a multidisciplinary international society of clinicians and scientists with an interest in vascular anomalies. It was formed based on international workshops for specialists interested in these disorders and officially founded in 1992, after its first International Workshop in 1990 (now called the 'International Congress') (7).

The ISSVA based its initial 1996 classification system on the established paradigm of stratifying vascular anomalies into proliferative vascular lesions, i.e., 'tumours' and relatively static 'vascular malformations' (7). This classification has been subsequently updated in 2014, 2018, and 2023 to include advances in clinical, pathologic, and genetic characteristics (Table 1.1) (https://www.issva.org/classification) (8).

Vascular tumours are characterised by endothelial cell hyperproliferation, and the ISSVA broadly categorises these as benign, intermediate, or malignant based on histological features and clinical behaviour (Table 1.2). The most common vascular tumours are infantile haemangiomas (IH) (Figure 1.2). The clinical diagnosis of IH is often based on a characteristic pattern of evolution. They are typically not present at birth, or the only indication may be a precursor lesion seen as a localised area of skin discolouration or telangiectasia (11). They then enter a proliferative phase, starting to grow at around 2 weeks to 2 months of life, typically peaking by 6 months of age. At this time, the lesion is usually raised and red in colour. The proliferative phase is followed by an involuting phase in which the lesion regresses spontaneously and decreases in size into late childhood. Finally, the fibrotic stage occurs, which is characterised by a residual scar (12).

In contrast, vascular malformations do not undergo abnormal cell turnover but, rather, result from localised errors in vascular morphogenesis that can affect arteries, veins, capillaries, and lymphatics (1). These are classified as fast-flow (Table 1.3), slow-flow (Table 1.4), and capillary (Table 1.5) (https://www.issva.org/classification). These are often present at birth but may be clinically silent and grow proportionally with the individual. They do not tend to regress.

Other distinct categories in which histology and clinical presentation do not allow clear distinction between tumour or malformation have been incorporated into the classification. These include complex lymphatic anomalies (Table 1.6), lymphoedema (Table 1.7), and developmental anomalies of named vessels (Table 1.8) (https://www.issva.org/classification).

The nomenclature in the ISSVA classification relies on a combination of clinical, radiological, and/or histopathologic features. This is extremely important and emphasises the multidisciplinary approach to the diagnosis and management of vascular anomalies. Whilst some lesions may have characteristic histological, immunohistochemical, or molecular features, the majority do not and, therefore, require interpretation in the context of all other factors present.

**TABLE 1.1**  Classification of vascular anomalies

| Vascular Tumours |
|---|
| Benign<br>Intermediate<br>Malignant |
| **Vascular Malformations** |
| Fast-flow<br>Slow-flow<br>Capillary |
| **Complex Lymphatic Anomalies** |
| **Lymphoedema** |
| **Developmental Anomalies of Named Vessels** |

**TABLE 1.2**  Vascular tumours

| Vascular Tumours | Causal Genes |
|---|---|
| **Benign** | |
| Infantile haemangioma (Figure 1.2) | |
| Congenital haemangioma<br>    Rapidly involuting (RICH)*<br>    Non-involuting (NICH)<br>    Partially involuting (PICH) | GNAQ/GNA11 |
| Pyogenic granuloma (Figure 1.3) | BRAF/RAS/GNA14 |
| Haemangiomas – other* | |
| **Intermediate** | |
| Tufted angioma | |
| Kaposiform haemangioendothelioma* (Figure 1.4) | GNA14 |
| Kaposi sarcoma | |
| MLT/CAT° | |
| Haemangioendotheliomas – other* | |
| **Malignant** | |
| Angiosarcoma | MYC |
| Epithelioid haemangioendothelioma | CAMTA1/TFE3 |

\*  May be associated with thrombocytopenia and/or consumptive coagulopathy.
˙  See reference for linked lists.
°  Multifocal lymphangioendotheliomatosis with thrombocytopenia/cutaneovisceral angiomatosis with thrombocytopenia.

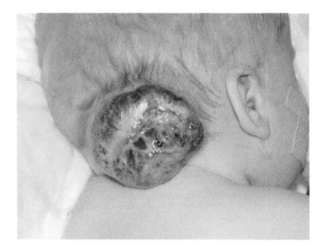

FIGURE 1.2 Ulcerated haemangioma of the neck at time of surgery. These lesions are painful and can bleed profusely.

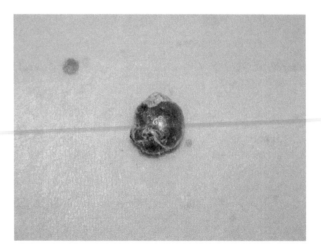

FIGURE 1.3 Pyogenic granuloma measuring 11 mm in diameter.

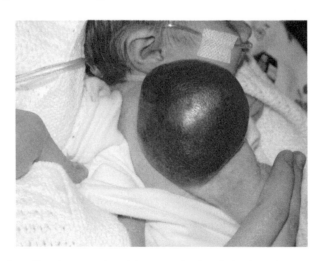

FIGURE 1.4 Baby with Kaposiform haemangioendothelioma (KHE) suffering from Kasabach–Merritt phenomenon (KMP), a clotting disorder resulting from the trapping of platelets within the vascular tumour.

**TABLE 1.3** Fast-flow vascular malformations

| Fast-Flow Vascular Malformation | Causal Genes |
|---|---|
| Arteriovenous malformation (AVM) | MAP2K1 |
| Arteriovenous fistula (AVF) | |
| Intra-muscular fast-flow vascular anomaly | MAP2K1 |
| CM of CM-AVM# | RASA1/EPHB4 |
| PTEN hamartoma of soft tissue (PHOST) | PTEN |

# Capillary malformations of capillary-arteriovenous malformations.

**TABLE 1.4** Slow-flow vascular malformations

| Slow-Flow Vascular Malformation | Causal Genes |
|---|---|
| Venous malformation (VM) | TEK (TIE2), PIK3CA |
| Lymphatic malformation (LM)* | PIK3CA, BRAF |
| Mixed slow-flow malformation (VLM) | PIK3CA PIK3R1 |
| Glomuvenous malformation (GVM) | Glomulin (GLMN) |
| Verrucous venous malformation (VVM) | MAP3K3 |
| Fibroadipose vascular anomaly (FAVA) | PIK3CA |
| Cerebral cavernoma | KRIT1, CCM2, PDCD10 |

* When associated with overgrowth, some of these lesions belong to the PIK3CA-related overgrowth spectrum.
Note: Some of these lesions may be associated with thrombocytopenia and/or consumptive coagulopathy.

**TABLE 1.5** Capillary vascular malformations (CM)

| Capillary Vascular Malformation | Causal Genes |
|---|---|
| Port-wine stain ('birthmark')# | GNAQ, GNB2, PTPN11, GNA11 |
| Diffuse capillary malformation with overgrowth (DCMO) | GNA11 |
| CM of megaencephaly-capillary malformation syndrome (MCAP) | PIK3CA |
| CMTC* | GNA11, AKT3 |
| Naevus simplex° | |

# Cutaneous and/or mucosal CM.
* Cutis marmorata telangiectatica congenita.
° Also 'salmon patch', 'angel kiss', and 'stork bite'.

**TABLE 1.6** Complex lymphatic anomalies

| Complex Lymphatic Anomaly | Causal Genes |
|---|---|
| Generalised lymphatic anomaly (GLA) | PIK3CA |
| Kaposiform lymphangiomatosis (KLA) | NRAS, CBL |
| Gorham–Stout disease (GSD) | KRAS |
| Central conducting lymphatic anomaly (CCLA) | ARAF, MDFIC, EPHB4 |

**TABLE 1.7** Lymphoedema*

| Lymphoedema | Causal Genes |
|---|---|
| **Primary** | |
| Isolated | FLT4 (VEGFR-3), VEGFC |
| Syndromic* | CCBE1, FOXC2, GJC2, GJA1, PTPN14, SOX18, HGF, KIF11, PTPN11, SOS1, IKBKG, GATA2, RASA1 |
| **Secondary** | |

\*  See https://www.issva.org/classification.

**TABLE 1.8** Developmental anomalies of named vessels

| Examples |
|---|
| Absent IVC |
| Aortic coarctation |
| Persistent embryological veins<br>    Lateral marginal<br>    Persistent sciatic |
| May–Thurner syndrome |
| Others |

*Source:* From (7).

# HISTOPATHOLOGICAL FEATURES

Where the clinical and/or radiological identification of a specific type of vascular lesion is not possible, the use of additional investigations may be necessary to reach a definitive diagnosis. Histopathological examination of a tissue biopsy sample, usually in conjunction with immunohistochemical stains and/or molecular techniques, can add useful information to aid diagnosis in a range of circumstances.

Histopathological examination of vascular tumours will generally demonstrate poorly circumscribed lesions composed of vessels, most often capillaries, with endothelial proliferations, while vascular malformations generally exhibit mature but dysplastic and/or abnormally organised blood vessels which infiltrate into surrounding tissues (see individual chapters for lesion-specific histological findings). Specific additional features may be present, depending on the precise type of lesion; for example, in arteriovenous malformations (AVMs) the elastic lamina is disrupted, and there is intimal fibrous thickening in arteries and arterialisation of veins, whereas in venous malformations, there are predominant abnormal and dysplastic venous channels (15).

In addition, special stains to highlight particular components along with immunohistochemical stains can be useful when examining such lesions, both to identify the type of endothelium present and also, in some circumstances, to help provide a specific diagnosis.

**TABLE 1.9**  Vascular malformations associated with other anomalies (7)

| Vascular Malformations Associated with Other Anomalies | Causal Genes |
|---|---|
| Klippel–Trenaunay syndrome:* CM + VM +/– LM + limb overgrowth | *PIK3CA* |
| Parkes Weber syndrome: CM + AVF + limb overgrowth | *RASA1* |
| Servelle–Martorell syndrome: limb VM + bone undergrowth | |
| Sturge–Weber syndrome: facial + leptomeningeal CM + eye anomalies +/– bone and/or soft tissue overgrowth | *GNAQ/GNA11/GNB2* |
| Limb CM + congenital non-progressive limb overgrowth | *GNA11* |
| Maffucci syndrome: VM +/– spindle-cell haemangioma + enchondroma | *IDH1/IDH2* |
| Macrocephaly – CM (M-CM/MCAP)* | *PIK3CA* |
| Microcephaly – CM (MICCAP) | *STAMBP* |
| CLOVES syndrome:* LM + VM + CM +/– AVM + lipomatous overgrowth | *PIK3CA* |
| Proteus syndrome: CM, VM, and/or LM + asymmetrical somatic overgrowth | *AKT1* |
| Bannayan–Riley–Ruvalcaba sd: AVM + VM + macrocephaly, lipomatous overgrowth | *PTEN* |
| CLAPO syndrome:* lower lip CM + face and neck LM + asymmetry and partial/generalised overgrowth | *PIK3CA* |

\* Belongs to the *PIK3CA*-related overgrowth spectrum.

For certain entities, tinctorial and immunohistochemical light microscopic examination may be diagnostic; for example, GLUT1 is a cytoplasmic endothelial stain expressed in IHs in all stages of evolution and is, therefore, a highly specific marker for this lesion in the appropriate clinical context (it is also strongly expressed in perineurium and in the placenta) but absent in congenital haemangiomas. Essentially infantile capillary haemangiomas are all GLUT1 positive. Almost all other vascular anomalies, haemangiomas, and vascular malformations are GLUT1 negative. Rarely, some other vascular lesions can show patchy or variable GLUT1 staining, for example, angiosarcoma (30% GLUT1 positive), epithelioid haemangioendothelioma (5% GLUT1 positive), and verrucous haemangiomas (VVM) (70% with some GLUT1 expression). Antibodies to CD31 (panendothelial cell marker) and CD34 (vascular endothelial marker) also stain the endothelial cells but are not specific for any particular lesion and are less useful in most circumstances. Other vascular immunostains, such as D2-40, PROX1, and VEGFR-3, can distinguish different types of endothelial cells – lymphatic type, for example – and may provide helpful diagnostic information.

It should be noted that interpretation of histopathological findings should always be in the context of the imaging and clinical features, including the specific type of biopsy (for example, a needle core biopsy may not be representative of the entire lesion), disease course (for example, histological features are different in proliferative versus regressive phases), and previous interventions (for example, sclerotherapy may be associated with specific iatrogenic features).

# IMAGING IN VASCULAR ANOMALIES

When vascular anomalies present as a cutaneous lesion with characteristic appearance, imaging is rarely necessary for diagnosis. However, deeper lesions will not discolour the skin and present as a very non-specific mass. Imaging provides useful diagnostic information in such cases and brings value when there are localised or systemic effects from the primary lesion. Imaging can demonstrate the extent of the lesion, its relationship to adjacent critical structures, and its vascular supply. Ultrasound (US), magnetic resonance imaging (MRI), and magnetic resonance angiography (MRA) are the usual modalities used for imaging vascular anomalies, though plain radiographs and computed tomography (CT) may have a role when bone is involved (13). All imaging modalities, however, can mislead if the imaging studies are not interpreted in the context of the clinical history and presentation. MRA has largely superseded the diagnostic role of conventional angiography, but conventional angiography plays a major role in high-flow lesions for which therapeutic intervention may be required (11,14).

---

## KEY MESSAGES

- The management of vascular anomalies has been significantly improved due to the introduction of the recent classifications.

- The agreement around nomenclature has improved understanding and communication between clinicians treating this group of conditions.

- Advances in the investigation, imaging, genetics, treatment modalities, and multidisciplinary care have led to significant benefits for patient outcomes.

# REFERENCES

1. Adams RH, Alitalo K. Molecular regulation of angiogenesis and lymphangiogenesis. *Nat Rev Mol Cell Biol.* 2007 Jun;8(6):464–78.
2. Hassanein AH, Mulliken JB, Fishman SJ, Greene AK. Evaluation of terminology for vascular anomalies in current literature. *Plast Reconstr Surg.* 2011 Jan;127(1):347–51.
3. Mulliken JB, Burrows PE, Fishman Steven J. *Mulliken and Young's Vascular Anomalies: Haemangiomas and Malformations* 2nd Edition. Oxford University Press; 2013. 22–39. ISBN: 9780195145052.
4. Virchow R. *Angioma in die Krankhaften Geschwülste.* Berlin: Verlag von August Hirschwald; 1863.
5. Mulliken, John BMD, Glowacki JPD. Hemangiomas and vascular malformations in infants and children: A classification based on endothelial characteristics. *Plast Reconstr Surg.* 1982;69(3):412–20.
6. Belov S. Classification of congenital vascular defects. *Int Angiol.* 1990;9(3):141–6.
7. International Society for the Study of Vascular Anomalies. ISSVA Classification of Vascular Anomalies ©2018 [Internet] [cited 2021 Aug 10]. Available from: issva.org/classification
8. International Society for the Study of Vascular Anomalies. ISSVA Classification of Vascular Anomalies 2023. [Internet] [cited 2023]. Available from http://issva.org/classification
9. Fletcher CDM, Unni K, Mertens F. World Health Organization classification of tumours. In *Pathology and Genetics of Tumours of Soft Tissue and Bone.* CDM Fletcher, KK Unni, F Mertens, editors. Lyon: IARC Press; 2002.
10. LeBoit Philip E, Burg Gunter, Weedon David, Sarasin Alain. Pathology and genetics of skin tumours. *World Health Organization Classification of Tumours.* PE LeBoit, G Burg, D Weedon, A Sarasin, editors. Lyon: IARC Press; 2005. ISBN 9789283224143.
11. Restrepo R, Palani R, Cervantes LF, Duarte AM, Amjad I, Altman NR. Hemangiomas revisited: The useful, the unusual and the new: Part 1: Overview and clinical and imaging characteristics. *Pediatr Radiol.* 2011 Jul;41(7):895–904.
12. Mattassi R, Loose DA, Vaghi M. *Hemangiomas and Vascular Malformations – An Atlas of Diagnosis and Treatment.* 2nd Edition. Milano: Springer Milan; 2015.
13. Restrepo R. Multimodality imaging of vascular anomalies. *Pediatr Radiol.* 2013 Mar;43(Suppl 1).
14. Dubois J, Alison M. Vascular anomalies: What a radiologist needs to know. *Pediatr Radiol.* 2010 Jun;40(6):895–905.
15. Patel RJ, Buch AC, Chandanwale SS, Kumar H. Role of histochemical stains in differentiating hemangioma and vascular malformation. *Indian J Dermatopathol Diagnostic Dermatology.* 2016;3(1):1.
16. Meijer-Jorna LB, Breugem CC, de Boer OJ, Ploegmakers JPM, van der Horst CMAM, van der Wal AC. Presence of a distinct neural component in congenital vascular malformations relates to the histological type and location of the lesion. *Hum Pathol.* 2009 Oct;40(10):1467–73.
17. Omar P, Sangueza LR. *Pathology of Vascular Skin Lesions: Clinicopathological Correlations.* Ivan Damjanov, editor. Totowa: Human Press Inc.; 2003. 7–15. ISBN: 9781592593606.

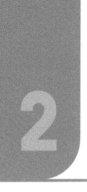

# 2 Genetics of Vascular Anomalies

Maanasa Polubothu and Jadesola Oyedepo

## INTRODUCTION

Vascular anomalies are caused by early defects in vascular development, secondary to genetic variants in critical genes in angiogenesis or growth pathways. Typically, they present at birth or in early childhood, but new lesions can appear over time. Over the past 10 years, we have come a long way in uncovering the genetic basis of many of these conditions (Figure 2.1). This has rapidly accelerated our understanding of the underlying pathogenesis of these lesions. The advent of next-generation sequencing has enabled the discovery of the genetic basis of these conditions. As many of these conditions are mosaic vascular disorders, the mutant allele load can be <1%, which is surprising given the often-dramatic phenotypes, but demonstrates the power of these classic oncogenic driver mutations.

In addition to adding to our understanding of the underlying pathophysiology, discovery of the underlying genetics of these conditions has opened the door to personalised medicine with existing licensed targeted therapies. By repurposing targeted inhibitors of the MAPK and PI3K pathway, there is a unique opportunity to take advantage of advances in precision cancer therapies to enable us to rapidly translate these genetic findings into medical treatment for these cohorts of children.

Establishing the genetic basis of vascular anomalies is also important to allow stratification of patients and may enable for better early prognostication and counselling for families. In the case of inherited germline vascular disorders, a genetic diagnosis in a child will help direct testing for family members and inform necessary surveillance for affected family members (Figure 2.2).

## INHERITED GERMLINE MUTATIONS

Inherited germline mutations are found in the hereditary haemorrhagic telangiectasia syndrome, CM-AVM syndrome, cerebral cavernous malformation, glomuvenous syndromes, and PTEN-hamartoma syndromes. Implicated genes are shown in Table 2.1. In general, these disorders are characterised by a germline mutation followed by a second somatic hit in lesional tissue conferring loss of function locally of a key protein. Initial assessment in suspected cases should include a detailed family history; and confirmed cases should be referred to a clinical geneticist to enable appropriate familial testing and genetic counselling.

## SOMATIC MUTATIONS

Somatic mutations are genetic variants that arise *in utero* during fetal development. This concept of genetic mosaicism allows for a broad phenotypic spectrum with the timing of the initial genetic event and the cell type in which it occurs, dictating the phenotype. They can be solitary or multifocal, and the same genetic change in different cell types can give rise to multiple types of vascular anomaly in the same patient due to the initial genetic event occurring in a progenitor cell capable of differentiation into different cell types. Somatic mutations in vascular anomalies are typically present at low levels in the sequenced tissue, often less than 5% of the sequenced reads. They are typically gain-of-function mutations leading to overactivation of critical growth pathways. As such, the majority of described somatic variants are oncogenes implicated in numerous human cancers. Somatic mutations described in vascular anomalies and tumours are outlined in Table 2.2.

Somatic Mutations

DOI: 10.1201/9781003257417-2

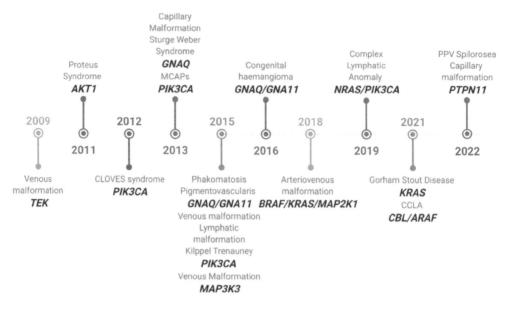

FIGURE 2.1 Timeline of genetic discovery in vascular anomalies.

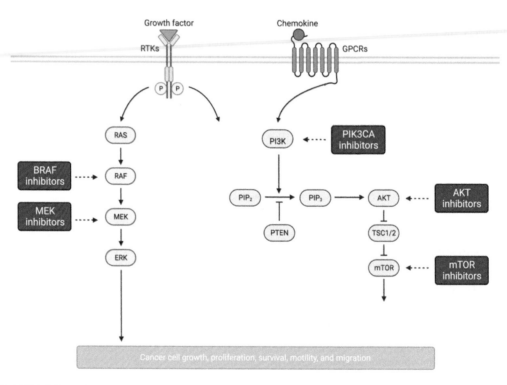

FIGURE 2.2 Key pathways implicated in vascular anomalies and potential targeted therapies.

**TABLE 2.1** Genetic causes of inherited vascular anomalies or syndromes

| Vascular Anomaly or Syndrome | Genetics |
|---|---|
| Hereditary haemorrhagic telangiectasia (HHT) | *ENG*<br>*ALK1*<br>*HHT3*<br>*HHT4*<br>*BMP9/GDF2* |
| CM-AVM syndrome | *RASA1*<br>*EPHB4* |
| PTEN-hamartoma tumour syndrome | *PTEN* |
| Cerebral cavernous malformation | *KRIT1*<br>*Malcavernin*<br>*PDCD10*<br>*CCM4* |
| Glomuvenous malformations | *GLMN (glomulin)* |

**TABLE 2.2** Genetic causes of somatic vascular malformations

| Vascular Anomaly | Genetics |
|---|---|
| Arteriovenous malformation | *KRAS*<br>*BRAF*<br>*MAP2K1* |
| Venous malformation | *TEK*<br>*PIK3CA* |
| Capillary malformation | *GNAQ*<br>*GNA11*<br>*PTPN11*<br>*PIK3CA*<br>*GNB2* |
| Congenital haemangioma | *GNAQ*<br>*GNA11*<br>*GNA14* |
| Glomuvenous malformations | *GLMN (glomulin)* |
| Lymphatic malformation | *BRAF*<br>*PIK3CA* |
| Complex lymphatic anomaly (Gorham–Stout, generalised lymphatic anomaly, kaposiform lymphatic anomaly, central collecting lymphatic anomaly) | *PIK3CA*<br>*NRAS*<br>*KRAS*<br>*ARAF*<br>*CBL*<br>(Also, germline recessive mutations in *EPHB4* and *MDFIC*) |
| Proteus syndrome | *AKT1* |
| *PIK3CA*-related overgrowth spectrum | *PIK3CA*<br>*PIK3R1* |
| Verrucous venous malformation | *MAP3K3* |

# APPROACH TO GENETIC TESTING FOR INHERITED GERMLINE VARIANTS

The approach to testing for germline inherited vascular disorders involves testing of DNA from blood or buccal mucosa. The hypothesis that underlies these conditions is a germline variant with a somatic second-hit in lesional tissue. As the initial germline variants are heterozygous in all tissues, standard sequencing approaches are sufficient for detection – for example, Sanger sequencing – although most modern diagnostic laboratories will utilise next-generation sequencing to enable rapid sequencing of all coding areas of candidate genes. High-depth sequencing of lesional tissue can demonstrate the second somatic hit, although this is not necessary for diagnosis.

# APPROACH TO GENETIC TESTING OF SOMATIC VARIANTS

Due to the mosaic nature of the majority of vascular anomalies, genetic testing using gold standard Sanger sequencing of leucocyte DNA will not demonstrate the causative genetic variant. DNA should be extracted directly from affected tissue and sequenced at a high depth, typically using next-generation sequencing or similar techniques that enable a high depth of sequencing, such as droplet digital PCR. Recent advances have shown that low-level mosaic genetic variants can also be demonstrated by sequencing of cell-free DNA derived from peripheral blood or cyst fluid in cases of lymphatic malformation. Whether these techniques are as reliable as direct sequencing of affected tissue is yet to be established; however, this approach is attractive, as it obviates the need for a biopsy which can be risky in certain lesions.

# OVERVIEW OF THE GENETICS OF VASCULAR ANOMALIES

## PIK3CA-RELATED OVERGROWTH SPECTRUM

Somatic activating mutations in the PI3K-AKT-mTOR pathway underlie a group of heterogeneous segmental overgrowth disorders and vascular anomalies. *PIK3CA*-related overgrowth spectrum (PROS) is an umbrella term describing the known and emerging clinical entities associated with somatic *PIK3CA*, including macrodactyly; congenital lipomatous overgrowth, vascular malformations, epidermal naevi, scoliosis/skeletal/spinal syndrome (CLOVES); fibroadipose hyperplasia or overgrowth (FAO); hemihyperplasia multiple lentigines (HHML); and related megalencephaly conditions (1). Many individuals present with overlapping features of syndromes previously thought to be clinically distinct. There is a broad phenotypic spectrum ranging from mild isolated overgrowth or minor vascular anomalies that do not interfere with function to severe multifocal extensive disease with extracutaneous organ involvement and haematological abnormalities.

## ARTERIOVENOUS MALFORMATIONS

Sporadic extracranial arteriovenous malformations are caused by somatic activating mutations in the genes *MAP2K1*, *KRAS*, and *BRAF* (2). Intracranial arteriovenous malformations are caused by the same genetic variants in *KRAS* (3). Clinically, these are challenging lesions, and knowledge of genotype in recent years has enabled targeted inhibition of the RAS-MAPK pathway with repurposed cancer therapies, with some early encouraging results (4, 5).

## CAPILLARY MALFORMATIONS

Capillary malformations are caused by somatic activating mutations in the genes *PIK3CA*, *GNA11* (6), *GNAQ* (7), *PTPN11* (8), and *GNB2* (9). Although subtle phenotypic clues can help differentiate the genetic basis of this group of vascular anomalies, genetic diagnosis in this group has important implications for prognosis, further imaging, and monitoring.

## VENOUS MALFORMATIONS

The majority of simple venous malformations are caused by somatic mutations in either *TEK* or *PIK3CA* (10, 11). Verrucous venous malformations have been shown to be due to mosaic mutations in *MAP3K3* (12). Glomuvenous malformations are caused by a germline mutation in the gene glomulin (*GLMN*) with a second somatic hit in lesional tissue (13).

## LYMPHATIC MALFORMATIONS

Solitary lymphatic malformations are caused by somatic activating mutations in *PIK3CA* and *BRAF* (14). Complex lymphatic anomaly, that is multifocal, can also be caused by mutations in *PIK3CA* and additionally *NRAS* (15), *CBL* (16), *ARAF* (17) and *KRAS* (18, 19), or germline variants in *EPHB4* (18, 19), and *MDFIC* (20). mTOR inhibition with sirolimus has been the mainstay of therapy for complex lymphatic anomaly for many years, but recent evidence in individual cases has demonstrated that targeted inhibition of the RAS/MAPK pathway can lead to dramatic remodelling of the lymphatic vasculature and improve symptoms (16, 17, 21).

## CM-AVM SYNDROME

CM-AVM syndrome is caused by a germline mutation in the genes *RASA1* and *EPHB4* with a second somatic genetic mutation demonstrated in the affected lesions of some patients (22–24). In early childhood, these lesions may be indistinguishable from capillary malformations, thus, an early genetic diagnosis in this cohort is critical to enable appropriate central nervous system (CNS) surveillance to identify the CNS vascular anomalies associated with this condition and to direct familial testing.

## BLUE RUBBER BLEB NAEVUS SYNDROME

Blue rubber bleb naevus syndrome (BRBNS) is a rare multisystem vascular disorder which presents at birth with multiple venous malformations. The clinical course may be complicated by severe gastrointestinal bleeding in cases in which the gut mucosa is involved. The genetic cause of BRBNS is recurrent double somatic mutations in *TEK* (25). The exact mechanism underlying this double somatic hit are unclear.

## PROTEUS SYNDROME

Proteus syndrome is an aggressive disorder of overgrowth caused by a recurrent somatic activating mutation in the gene *AKT1* (26). It is characterised by aggressive disproportionate overgrowth, leading to severe deformity, multiple vascular anomalies and other cutaneous naevi, tumours, and clotting abnormalities. Prognosis is poor with morbidity secondary to restrictive lung disease frequently seen in the second to third decade (27). Often at birth, these patients are indistinguishable from those with other causes of overgrowth which follow a more indolent course. Early genotyping is critical in this cohort to manage the complex multisystem involvement and determine eligibility for targeted therapies, with recent evidence emerging that pan-AKT inhibitors can limit aggressive overgrowth in childhood (28, 29).

## CONGENITAL HAEMANGIOMA

Congenital haemangiomas are vascular tumours present at birth which most commonly involute in the first 14 months of life but can cause severe morbidity in the neonatal period secondary to cardiac failure owing to the high-flow nature of the most severe tumours. They are caused by somatic activating mutations in *GNAQ*, *GNA11*, and *GNA14*.

# TARGETED MEDICAL THERAPIES FOR VASCULAR ANOMALIES

In recent years, the use of targeted therapies for vascular anomalies has transformed the therapeutic landscape for these largely incurable conditions. The majority of these drugs were devised as cancer therapies and can have significant side effects, including immunosuppression. For vascular anomalies, unlike with most cancers, treatment may have to be lifelong. Thus, the decision to commence medical therapy should be the consensus of a multidisciplinary vascular anomalies team, and treatment should be monitored closely by an experienced paediatrician or oncologist with experience using these drugs.

## PI3K-AKT-mTOR PATHWAY INHIBITION

Sirolimus, an mTOR, inhibitor has been used for more than ten years in a number of vascular anomalies, including lymphatic anomalies, PROS, and PHOST (30–32). More recently, alpelisib, a novel PI3Kα inhibitor, has shown efficacy in *PIK3CA*-related overgrowth syndromes and isolated venous malformations secondary to *TEK* mutations (33, 34). The pan-AKT inhibitor miransertib has been used in patients with Proteus syndrome and has been shown to limit the aggressive skeletal overgrowth and reduce tumour volume in some patients (28).

## RAS-RAF-MAPK PATHWAY INHIBITION

MEK inhibition using, most commonly, trametinib has recently been shown to be an effective treatment for RAS-MAPK pathway complex lymphatic anomaly with reported rapid remodelling of the lymphatic system (17, 21) and RAS-MAPK pathway arteriovenous malformations with reduction in volume and flow (4, 5).

As highlighted by Mulliken in his foreword, the field of molecular genetics will be the avenue that develops our understanding and ability to treat vascular anomalies in the future.

---

### KEY MESSAGES

* Sporadic vascular anomalies and overgrowth syndromes are caused by somatic mutations in genes encoding key proteins in growth-signalling pathways, most often involving the PI3K-AKT-mTOR or RAS-RAF-MAPK signalling pathways.

* Genetic testing for these conditions requires testing of DNA extracted directly from affected tissue sequenced at high depth.

* Hereditary syndromes affecting the vasculature are caused by germline mutations in genes encoding key proteins in growth-signalling or angiogenesis pathways.

* Genetic testing for these conditions can be performed on blood/buccal DNA using standard sequencing methods to demonstrate causative heterozygous variants.

* In the case of inherited germline vascular disorders, a genetic diagnosis in a child will help direct testing for family members – these patients and their families should be referred to a clinical geneticist for genetic counselling and screening.

* Targeted medical therapies, many of which are drugs developed for cancer and repurposed for vascular anomalies and overgrowth, have transformed the prospects for some children with severe disease not amenable to surgical/radiological intervention.

* Routine genotyping of all patients with either inherited or sporadic vascular anomalies is, thus, recommended when it is safe, to inform prognosis, risk of transmission to offspring, and determine eligibility for novel targeted therapies.

---

# REFERENCES

1. Keppler-Noreuil, K.M., Rios, J.J., Parker, V.E., Semple, R.K., Lindhurst, M.J., Sapp, J.C., Alomari, A., Ezaki, M., Dobyns, W., and Biesecker, L.G. (2015). *PIK3CA*-related overgrowth spectrum (PROS): Diagnostic and testing eligibility criteria, differential diagnosis, and evaluation. *American Journal of Medical Genetics Part A* 167A, 287–295.
2. Al-Olabi, L., Polubothu, S., Dowsett, K., Andrews, K.A., Stadnik, P., Joseph, A.P., Knox, R., Pittman, A., Clark, G., Baird, W., et al. (2018). Mosaic RAS/MAPK variants cause sporadic vascular malformations which respond to targeted therapy. *Journal of Clinical Investigation* 128(11), 5185. doi: 10.1172/JCI124649.
3. Nikolaev, S.I., Vetiska, S., Bonilla, X., Boudreau, E., Jauhiainen, S., Rezai Jahromi, B., Khyzha, N., DiStefano, P.V., Suutarinen, S., Kiehl, T.-R., et al. (2018). Somatic activating KRAS mutations in arteriovenous malformations of the brain. *New England Journal of Medicine* 378, 250–261.
4. Edwards, E.A., Phelps, A.S., Cooke, D., Frieden, I.J., Zapala, M.A., Fullerton, H.J., and Shimano, K.A. (2020). Monitoring arteriovenous malformation response to genotype-targeted therapy. *Pediatrics* 146, e20193206. doi: 10.1542/peds.2019-3206.
5. Lekwuttikarn, R., Lim, Y.H., Admani, S., Choate, K.A., and Teng, J.M.C. (2019). Genotype-guided medical treatment of an arteriovenous malformation in a child. *JAMA Dermatology* 155, 256–257.
6. Thomas, A.C., Zeng, Z., Riviere, J.B., O'Shaughnessy, R., Al-Olabi, L., St-Onge, J., Atherton, D.J., Aubert, H., Bagazgoitia, L., Barbarot, S., et al. (2016). Mosaic activating mutations in GNA11 and GNAQ are associated with phakomatosis pigmentovascularis and extensive dermal melanocytosis. *Journal of Investigative Dermatology* 136(4), 770–778.
7. Shirley, M.D., Tang, H., Gallione, C.J., Baugher, J.D., Frelin, L.P., Cohen, B., North, P.E., Marchuk, D.A., Comi, A.M., and Pevsner, J. (2013). Sturge-Weber syndrome and port-wine stains caused by somatic mutation in GNAQ. *New England Journal of Medicine* 368, 1971–1979.
8. Polubothu, S., Bender, N., Muthiah, S., Zecchin, D., Demetriou, C., Martin, S.B., Malhotra, S., Travnickova, J., Zeng, Z., Böhm, M., et al. (2022). PTPN11 mosaicism causes a spectrum of pigmentary and vascular neurocutaneous disorders and predisposes to melanoma. *Journal of Investigative Dermatology* 143(6), 1042–1051. doi: 10.1016/j.jid.2022.09.661.
9. Fjær, R., Marciniak, K., Sundnes, O., Hjorthaug, H., Sheng, Y., Hammarström, C., Sitek, J.C., Vigeland, M.D., Backe, P.H., Øye, A.M., et al. (2021). A novel somatic mutation in GNB2 provides new insights to the pathogenesis of Sturge-Weber syndrome. *Human Molecular Genetics* 30, 1919–1931.

10. Limaye, N., Wouters, V., Uebelhoer, M., Tuominen, M., Wirkkala, R., Mulliken, J.B., Eklund, L., Boon, L.M., and Vikkula, M. (2009). Somatic mutations in angiopoietin receptor gene TEK cause solitary and multiple sporadic venous malformations. *Nature Genetics* 41, 118–124.
11. Castillo, S.D., Tzouanacou, E., Zaw-Thin, M., Berenjeno, I.M., Parker, V.E., Chivite, I., Mila-Guasch, M., Pearce, W., Solomon, I., Angulo-Urarte, A., et al. (2016). Somatic activating mutations in *PIK3CA* cause sporadic venous malformations in mice and humans. *Science Translational Medicine* 8, 332ra343.
12. Couto, J.A., Vivero, M.P., Kozakewich, H.P., Taghinia, A.H., Mulliken, J.B., Warman, M.L., and Greene, A.K. (2015). A somatic MAP3K3 mutation is associated with verrucous venous malformation. *American Journal of Human Genetics* 96, 480–486.
13. Brouillard, P., Boon, L.M., Mulliken, J.B., Enjolras, O., Ghassibé, M., Warman, M.L., Tan, O.T., Olsen, B.R., and Vikkula, M. (2002). Mutations in a novel factor, glomulin, are responsible for glomuvenous malformations ("glomangiomas"). *American Journal of Human Genetics* 70, 866–874.
14. Zenner, K., Jensen, D.M., Dmyterko, V., Shivaram, G.M., Myers, C.T., Paschal, C.R., Rudzinski, E.R., Pham, M.M., Cheng, V.C., Manning, S.C., et al. (2022). Somatic activating BRAF variants cause isolated lymphatic malformations. *Human Genetics and Genomics Advances* 3, 100101.
15. Barclay, S.F., Inman, K.W., Luks, V.L., McIntyre, J.B., Al-Ibraheemi, A., Church, A.J., Perez-Atayde, A.R., Mangray, S., Jeng, M., Kreimer, S.R., et al. (2019). A somatic activating NRAS variant associated with kaposiform lymphangiomatosis. *Genetics in Medicine* 21, 1517–1524.
16. Foster, J.B., Li, D., March, M.E., Sheppard, S.E., Adams, D.M., Hakonarson, H., and Dori, Y. (2020). Kaposiform lymphangiomatosis effectively treated with MEK inhibition. *EMBO Molecular Medicine* 12, e12324.
17. Li, D., March, M.E., Gutierrez-Uzquiza, A., Kao, C., Seiler, C., Pinto, E., Matsuoka, L.S., Battig, M.R., Bhoj, E.J., Wenger, T.L., et al. (2019). ARAF recurrent mutation causes central conducting lymphatic anomaly treatable with a MEK inhibitor. *Nature Medicine* 25, 1116–1122.
18. Nozawa, A., Ozeki, M., Niihori, T., Suzui, N., Miyazaki, T., and Aoki, Y. (2020). A somatic activating KRAS variant identified in an affected lesion of a patient with Gorham-Stout disease. *Journal of Human Genetics* 65, 995–1001.
19. Lacasta-Plasin, C., Martinez-Glez, V., Rodriguez-Laguna, L., Cervantes-Pardo, A., Martinez-Menchon, T., Sanchez-Jimenez, R., and Campos-Dominguez, M. (2021). KRAS mutation identified in a patient with melorheostosis and extended lymphangiomatosis treated with sirolimus and trametinib. *Clinical Genetics* 100, 484–485.
20. Byrne, A.B., Brouillard, P., Sutton, D.L., Kazenwadel, J., Montazaribarforoushi, S., Secker, G.A., Oszmiana, A., Babic, M., Betterman, K.L., Brautigan, P.J., et al. (2022). Pathogenic variants in MDFIC cause recessive central conducting lymphatic anomaly with lymphedema. *Science Translational Medicine* 14, eabm4869.
21. Chowers, G., Abebe-Campino, G., Golan, H., Vivante, A., Greenberger, S., Soudack, M., Barkai, G., Fox-Fisher, I., Li, D., March, M., et al. (2022). Treatment of severe kaposiform lymphangiomatosis positive for NRAS mutation by MEK inhibition. *Pediatr Research.* doi: 10.1038/s41390-022-01986-0.
22. Eerola, I., Boon, L.M., Mulliken, J.B., Burrows, P.E., Dompmartin, A., Watanabe, S., Vanwijck, R., and Vikkula, M. (2003). Capillary malformation-arteriovenous malformation, a new clinical and genetic disorder caused by RASA1 mutations. *American Journal of Human Genetics* 73, 1240–1249.
23. Amyere, M., Revencu, N., Helaers, R., Pairet, E., Baselga, E., Cordisco, M., Chung, W., Dubois, J., Lacour, J.P., Martorell, L., et al. (2017). Germline loss-of-function mutations in EPHB4 cause a second form of capillary malformation-arteriovenous malformation (CM-AVM2) deregulating RAS-MAPK signaling. *Circulation* 136, 1037–1048.
24. Lapinski, P.E., Doosti, A., Salato, V., North, P., Burrows, P.E., and King, P.D. (2018). Somatic second hit mutation of RASA1 in vascular endothelial cells in capillary malformation-arteriovenous malformation. *European Journal of Medical Genetics* 61, 11–16.
25. Soblet, J., Kangas, J., Natynki, M., Mendola, A., Helaers, R., Uebelhoer, M., Kaakinen, M., Cordisco, M., Dompmartin, A., Enjolras, O., et al. (2017). Blue rubber bleb nevus (BRBN) syndrome is caused by somatic TEK (TIE2) mutations. *Journal of Investigative Dermatology* 137, 207–216.
26. Lindhurst, M.J., Sapp, J.C., Teer, J.K., Johnston, J.J., Finn, E.M., Peters, K., Turner, J., Cannons, J.L., Bick, D., Blakemore, L., et al. (2011). A mosaic activating mutation in AKT1 associated with the Proteus syndrome. *New England Journal of Medicine* 365, 611–619.
27. Sapp, J.C., Hu, L., Zhao, J., Gruber, A., Schwartz, B., Ferrari, D., and Biesecker Md, L.G. (2017). Quantifying survival in patients with Proteus syndrome. *Genetics in Medicine* 19, 1376–1379.
28. Ours, C.A., Sapp, J.C., Hodges, M.B., de Moya, A.J., and Biesecker, L.G. (2021). Case report: Five-year experience of AKT inhibition with miransertib (MK-7075) in an individual with Proteus syndrome. *Cold Spring Harb Mol Case Stud* 7, a006134. doi: 10.1101/mcs.a006134.
29. Leoni, C., Gullo, G., Resta, N., Fagotti, A., Onesimo, R., Schwartz, B., Kazakin, J., Abbadessa, G., Crown, J., Collins, C.D., et al. (2019). First evidence of a therapeutic effect of miransertib in a teenager with Proteus syndrome and ovarian carcinoma. *American Journal of Medical Genetics Part A* 179, 1319–1324.
30. Adams, D.M., Trenor, C.C., 3rd, Hammill, A.M., Vinks, A.A., Patel, M.N., Chaudry, G., Wentzel, M.S., Mobberley-Schuman, P.S., Campbell, L.M., Brookbank, C., et al. (2016). Efficacy and safety of sirolimus in the treatment of complicated vascular anomalies. *Pediatrics* 137, e20153257.
31. Parker, V.E.R., Keppler-Noreuil, K.M., Faivre, L., Luu, M., Oden, N.L., De Silva, L., Sapp, J.C., Andrews, K., Bardou, M., Chen, K.Y., et al. (2019). Safety and efficacy of low-dose sirolimus in the PIK3CA-related overgrowth spectrum. *Genetics in Medicine* 21, 1189–1198.
32. Komiya, T., Blumenthal, G.M., DeChowdhury, R., Fioravanti, S., Ballas, M.S., Morris, J., Hornyak, T.J., Wank, S., Hewitt, S.M., Morrow, B., et al. (2019). A pilot study of sirolimus in subjects with Cowden syndrome or other syndromes characterized by germline mutations in PTEN. *Oncologist* 24, 1510-e1265.
33. Venot, Q., Blanc, T., Rabia, S.H., Berteloot, L., Ladraa, S., Duong, J.P., Blanc, E., Johnson, S.C., Hoguin, C., Boccara, O., et al. (2018). Targeted therapy in patients with *PIK3CA*-related overgrowth syndrome. *Nature* 558, 540–546.
34. Remy, A., Tran, T.H., Dubois, J., Gavra, P., Lapointe, C., Winikoff, R., Facundo, G.B., Théorêt, Y., and Kleiber, N. (2022). Repurposing alpelisib, an anti-cancer drug, for the treatment of severe TIE2-mutated venous malformations: Preliminary pharmacokinetics and pharmacodynamic data. *Pediatr Blood Cancer* 69, e29897.

# Haematology 3

Mary Mathias

## INTRODUCTION

The vast majority of children with vascular anomalies will never need any haematological investigations or input, but there are two situations in which it is vital that a haematologist is involved.

- The urgent management of disseminated intravascular coagulation in the context of patients with kaposiform haemangioendotheliomas (KHE) (Figure 3.1) or tufted angiomas (TA) (Figure 3.2).
- The chronic management of coagulopathy in patients with extensive slow-flow venous malformations, including blue rubber bleb naevus syndrome (Figure 3.3).

These two groups of pathologies can lead to haemostatic abnormalities which appear superficially similar and are often confused but require different management strategies. The first may present as a haematological emergency, sometimes even before the vascular malformation is diagnosed, whereas the second provides a longer term challenge for the patient and all the clinicians involved. Recognising the differences in aetiology in the haemostatic abnormalities in these two groups and understanding the possible haematological interventions is made easier by an understanding of the normal processes of coagulation.

## NORMAL HAEMOSTASIS

The physiology of normal haemostasis can be inhospitable to those who rarely need to engage with it. The following will not provide state of the art explanations of how blood should clot but is intended to give an overview of the balancing act our bodies achieve in order to provide prompt and anatomically specific cessation of bleeding whilst, at the same time, preventing widespread thrombosis.

The three factors necessary for normal haemostasis are:

1. Normal blood flow
2. Normal vascular endothelium
3. Normal proportions of procoagulant and anticoagulant proteins and a normal quantity and functioning of blood cells involved in haemostasis, principally platelets

Whilst it is easier to separate these factors conceptually and in investigations, it is vital to remember that they are part of a whole and that while we can, for instance, measure the circulating level of a coagulation protein relatively easily, we are doing that by taking a sample of blood from the child, anticoagulating that sample until it reaches the laboratory and then reversing the anticoagulation in order to allow a clot to form in a static model of haemostasis, far from the child's blood vessel or their platelets. It gives us some clues about what is happening *in vivo* but not the entire picture.

The historical models of haemostasis focused on pathways of activation of the clotting factors via the 'intrinsic' and 'extrinsic' pathways: the first in which thrombin generation is triggered by activation of contact factors such as factor XII and the second being triggered by the exposure of tissue factor (tF) at the site of vessel wall damage. These models were again a reflection of our ability as doctors and

DOI: 10.1201/9781003257417-3

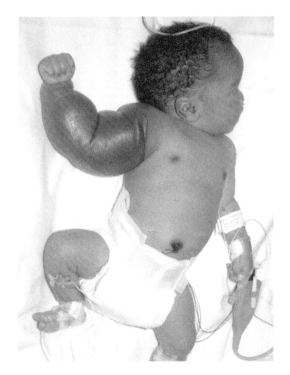

FIGURE 3.1 A newborn child with a kaposiform haemangioendotheliomas (KHE) lesion of the right upper limb.

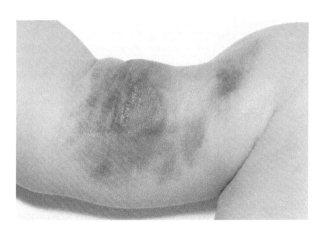

FIGURE 3.2 Tufted angioma of the right upper arm of a 5-month-old child.

scientists to analyse the steps involved in a laboratory (contact factors being those that are activated by contact with a glass surface). The current recognition that both 'arms' of the 'clotting cascade' are integrated and coexistent is a much better fit both physiologically and pathologically.

It is important to be aware that the normal levels of many of the coagulation proteins are age dependent and that results should be interpreted with a knowledge of age-appropriate normal ranges.

Thrombin (or factor IIa) is the critical centre of the haemostatic process, as once it is generated, it both allows amplification of further thrombin generation and, at the same time, triggers the pathways that limit a clot to the site of vessel injury and prevents propagation. It is said to be 'the author of its own destruction' for this reason.

Our current understanding is that exposed tF at the site of endothelial damage binds with factor X (FX) and generates thrombin. The tF/FX complex is normally rapidly 'turned off' by tF pathway

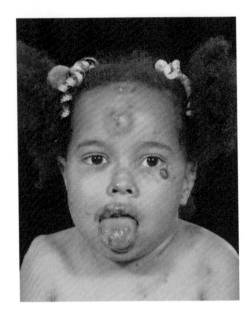

FIGURE 3.3 Extensive blue rubber bleb naevus syndrome (BRBNS) in a 4-year-old girl.

inhibitor. The modest amount of thrombin initially generated then brings about a thrombin 'burst' with a massive positive feedback amplification loop. It also converts soluble fibrinogen to insoluble fibrin and facilitates cross-linking of the fibrin by factor XIII (FXIII), resulting in a stable, lysis-resistant clot. In addition to fibrin, the clot is composed of platelets, red blood cells, and white blood cells.

Thrombin also brings about the activation of protein C (which down-regulates the FVIII/V complex and prevents ongoing amplification of the thrombin burst) and antithrombin, which inhibits thrombin. Circulating plasminogen binds to the clot and is converted to plasmin, which breaks down fibrin into its degradation products, amongst which are D dimers.

Whilst the coagulation proteins interact to create stable, cross-linked fibrin, platelets are also in parallel playing a vital role in clot formation. When platelets, marginalised at the periphery of a blood vessel, come in contact with damaged endothelium and exposed collagen, they adhere to the vessel wall, with von Willebrand factor acting as an adhesive. They undergo shape change, which increases their surface area and provides a negatively charged phospholipid membrane on which many of the protein interactions can take place. Platelet adhesion is especially promoted in vessels with high sheer stress, such as those of smaller calibre or those containing high-flow rates.

Coagulation 'screening tests' reflect different elements of the coagulation proteins involved in haemostasis. They are able to identify a gross abnormality but are not helpful in picking up subtle trends. A screen typically includes:

- Prothrombin time (PT)
- Activated partial thromboplastin time (APTT)
- Fibrinogen (this may either be derived from the PT or the fibrinogen). If the fibrinogen level falls below the lower limit of normal, the PT and APTT will gradually start to prolong, as these tests are ultimately reliant on fibrin formation

Additional haemostatic tests which may be helpful in children with vascular anomalies include:

- Individual clotting factor assays, including FXIII
- D-dimer level

# DISSEMINATED INTRAVASCULAR COAGULATION IN VASCULAR ANOMALIES

In both KHE/TA and venous malformations, there are fundamental disturbances in blood flow, the vascular endothelium (1), and as a result, the composition of some of the pro- and anticoagulant proteins. Small thrombi occur within the body of the vascular anomaly, leading to significant consumption of coagulation proteins and, in some cases, a fall in platelets and haemoglobin, with the classical features of a microangiopathic haemolytic anaemia (MAHA) on the blood film (2). When the trigger for MAHA is systemic (for example, in sepsis), the thrombi and consumption occur throughout the body and are termed disseminated intravascular coagulation (DIC). With vascular anomalies, there is the very singular situation that the pathological process of thrombus generation is localised to the body of the lesion itself. The term *localised* intravascular coagulation has, therefore, been coined, but, of course, any imbalance in coagulation proteins or the platelet count is not localised to the vascular anomaly because of the systemic circulation of the blood. Thus, in a child with a coagulopathy caused by their vascular anomaly, surgery at the site of the lesion would be associated with a bleeding risk but so would surgery at a distant site (3, 4).

# KASABACH–MERRITT PHENOMENON (KMP)

Kasabach–Merritt phenomenon (KMP), sometimes referred to as Kasabach–Merritt syndrome (KMS), describes a coagulopathy caused by certain rapidly growing vascular tumours, specifically KHE and, less commonly, TA. It is very rare but may present as a haematological emergency in the first few days of life. It comprises very low platelet counts (often $<10 \times 10^9/L$), low fibrinogen levels, and anaemia. The process is aggressive and can be life-threatening. Where the KHE or TA involves the skin and is clinically apparent, the diagnosis can be made rapidly, but if the lesion is deep seated, the only initial abnormality may be the abnormal haematological results. In the case of a neonate with DIC and no other apparent cause, this diagnosis must always be considered and ruled out with imaging.

The treatment, as with all DIC, is of the underlying condition (see Chapter 6), but given the extreme derangement of coagulation, it is sometimes necessary to provide temporary support with blood products. Current guidance would be to replace platelets in a bleeding child if the count is below $25 \times 10^9/L$ (5). However, in the context of KMP, there is a school of thought that it is best to avoid transfusion with platelets or blood if possible in the belief that this may 'add fuel to the fire' of the consumptive process. The evidence base is very small, and the possible risk of exacerbating the DIC must be balanced against the risk of bleeding (most significantly, intracerebral bleeding) in a neonate. Figure 3.4 shows a case of KMP responding to multiple treatment modalities with a recovering platelet count.

The DIC in KMP, whilst life-threatening and requiring urgent management in a centre with a multidisciplinary team familiar with the treatment and support needed, can respond to therapy within a few weeks. If this is successful, the child's coagulopathy will resolve. This is in direct contrast to children and young adults with venous malformations whose coagulopathy is often life-long and may worsen with age.

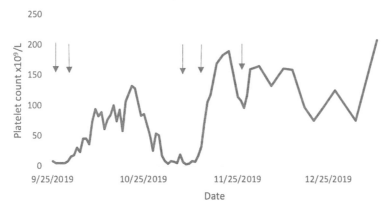

FIGURE 3.4 Platelet response to therapy in a case of Kasabach-Merritt phenomenon. Sirolimus was given throughout the time course along with pulses of methylprednisolone and then prednisolone. Arrows denote doses of vincristine.

# VENOUS MALFORMATIONS

This description encompasses a number of histological and phenotypic variations of venous malformation (VM) described in other chapters of this book. It may be that, with increasingly detailed understanding of the histological and genetic variation in this group of patients, it will be possible to predict which individuals will have the most severe coagulopathies. However, our experience suggests that the level of haematological abnormality is most obviously correlated with the 'volume' of the VM in relation to the size of the child. For example, a VM affecting part of the forearm in isolation may be associated with a modest elevation in the D-dimer level but will not be associated with significant consumptive coagulopathy. In contrast, a child with an extensive VM affecting the whole of one leg would be likely to have a significant coagulopathy. It is our observation, and that of other groups, that the coagulopathy in VM patients can worsen with age, which presumably is also a reflection of an increased volume of involved tissue as the patient grows (6).

There is a typical progressive sequence of haemostatic abnormality in this group of patients, described in Figure 3.5.

- The initial 'signal' is an elevation in the D-dimer level. This reflects an increase in clot formation and turnover as fibrin degradation products increase in the circulation. Elevated D-dimers are known to affect fibrinogen function, and this may contribute to falling functional fibrinogen levels.
- The next stage is a gradual fall in the fibrinogen level, followed by a gradual rise in the PT and APTT values. As mentioned above, because the PT and APTT assays are dependent on clot formation in the analyser, a reduction in fibrinogen levels has an impact on the results. In other words, if there is reduced fibrinogen present, clot formation will be impaired, and the PT and APTT would be prolonged, even if the other clotting factors were within normal limits.
- When the fibrinogen is below the lower limit of the normal range, the FXIII level will also start to fall; this can only be detected with a FXIII assay (7).
- Ultimately, the platelet count will start to fall if the volume of the VM is large enough (8).

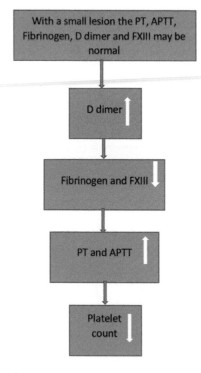

FIGURE 3.5 Progression of haemostatic test abnormalities over time in some patients with a venous malformation. The progression of coagulopathy is likely to occur over many years. PT: prothrombin time, APTT: activated partial thromboplastin time.

It is almost inevitable that even a small VM will be associated with a rise in D dimers; however, only a handful of children with very extensive malformations will progress to thrombocytopenia as a result of chronic DIC. The age-related progressive coagulopathy is demonstrated in Figure 3.6, showing that there is a gradual worsening of all parameters, but this can take many years.

Measurement of individual coagulation factors in a patient with DIC will generally demonstrate a global reduction in levels; however, in DIC triggered by VMs, there appears to be a more unusual

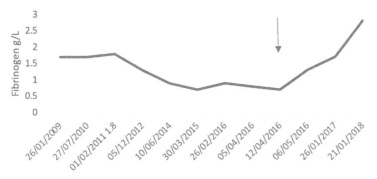

Fibrinogen levels in a patient with an extensive
VM before and after debulking surgery

FIGURE 3.6 Fibrinogen levels in a patient with an extensive VM pre- and post-debulking surgery. Arrow denotes day of debulking surgery. The patient was treated with low molecular weight heparin before and after the surgery and with fibrinogen concentrate around the surgical procedure. This demonstrates the slow progressive decline in fibrinogen prior to surgery and return to normal levels after debulking of the VM.

imbalance. In some instances, the clotting factors with the shorter half-lives, such as FVII and V, are reduced a little, but there is a very marked and disproportionate reduction in FXIII in children for whom the fibrinogen levels have fallen below the lower end of the normal range for age.

# MANAGEMENT OF CHRONIC DIC ASSOCIATED WITH VMs

The treatment for any cause of DIC is of the precipitating pathology. In many situations, such as sepsis or major haemorrhage, this is relatively straight forward. The chronic DIC caused by VMs is not easily solved. If the volume of the lesion can be significantly reduced surgically, then an improvement in, or resolution of, the coagulation abnormalities is possible. In the majority of cases in which there is severe coagulopathy, however, extensive surgical resection is not possible or carries too high a risk in the presence of such a significant coagulopathy. Medical management, such as treatment with sirolimus, can also have a positive effect on DIC in those children for whom it is indicated, but systemic therapy may not be advised in all patients or may not be effective (9).

From a haematological perspective, this leaves management of the DIC itself as the only option. This can be divided into (a) medical treatment to 'break the cycle' of DIC and (b) support with blood products in the face of bleeding or when an invasive procedure is planned.

## ANTICOAGULATION WITH LOW MOLECULAR WEIGHT HEPARIN

The concept of treating DIC with heparin is long standing, and it has been assessed in numerous clinical trials in the intensive care setting (2). The rationale is that preventing microthrombus formation with heparin will subsequently prevent the depletion of clotting factors and thrombocytopenia.

Use of this approach in VM was described in 2002 by Mazoyer (10) as being the only effective medical treatment for DIC in this context. The starting dose of low molecular weight heparin (LMWH), in our experience, should be dependent on the severity of the DIC in the individual; a child with a fibrinogen level of 0.3 g/L (lower limit of normal 1.7 g/L) should be started at a low dose which can then be increased, if necessary, as the fibrinogen improves. We typically start with a dose lower than the standard dose for prophylactic use.

Correction of, or at least improvement in, DIC can begin within a few days of commencing LMWH, but we aim to start it approximately 2 weeks prior to a planned intervention and to continue its post-intervention until healing is complete. This maximises the chance of normal wound healing without infection.

## OTHER SUPPORTIVE MEASURES AROUND EPISODES OF BLEEDING OR SURGICAL INTERVENTION

If the fibrinogen still remains below the lower limit of normal at the time of a surgical intervention, blood product support is likely to be needed. This is not generally the case for sclerotherapy, in which the haemostatic challenge is minimal (percutaneous access of the VM) and not usually associated with significant bleeding as long as firm pressure is applied at the time the needle is removed.

The intensity and duration of fibrinogen support should be proportionate to the nature of the surgery. For example, a tonsillectomy, which is one of the most haemostatically challenging procedures, will require normal or near normal coagulation for 10–14 days, whereas removal of an in-growing toenail would not need such intense support. Fibrinogen support, ideally, should be in the form of fibrinogen concentrate. The rationale behind this is that it supports fibrinogen but does not lead to an increase in FVIII and von Willebrand factor, both of which are present in cryoprecipitate; it can be given in a smaller volume; it is derived from pooled plasma fractionation; and the manufacturing process will involve viral inactivation steps.

FXIII may also be required if it remains significantly below the normal range at the time of surgery. This can be replaced with FXIII concentrate if that is available, and it is also present in cryoprecipitate, if this is the only source of fibrinogen available. FXIII may also be present as a constituent of fibrinogen concentrate (this varies between products).

The use of tranexamic acid around the time of episodes of bleeding or surgical interventions in a patient with DIC is controversial. Tranexamic acid works by binding to stable, cross-linked fibrin and slowing down the rate at which this is degraded by plasmin. In the majority of situations, tranexamic acid would be avoided because of concern about the possibility of increasing thrombotic risk. Data from the CRASH studies has improved our understanding of the efficacy and safety of tranexamic in many clinical scenarios, including acute trauma and obstetric haemorrhage (11). In children with VMs and bleeding or major surgery, we have found tranexamic acid both effective and safe.

---

**SUPPORT FOR BLEEDING OR SURGERY IN THE PRESENCE OF DIC ASSOCIATED WITH VMs (See Figure 3.7)**

- Start low-dose LMWH at least 14 days prior to a planned procedure, if possible.
- Repeat FBC, coagulation screen, and FXIII level the day prior to the procedure.
- Give the last dose of LMWH 24–48 hours prior to the procedure.
- If fibrinogen is below normal range, support with fibrinogen concentrate and FXIII concentrate if necessary.
- If platelets are <100 × 10$^9$/L at the time of the procedure, consider transfusion.
- Start tranexamic acid the day before the procedure.
- Monitor coagulation during (if procedure is long) and after the procedure, and continue to support with blood products when necessary.
- Restart low-dose LMWH after the procedure when haemostasis is secure, after discussion with the surgical team, and continue until wound healing is complete along with tranexamic acid.

---

For some children/young adults with severe DIC associated with recurrent painful clots and bleeding symptoms, long-term use of LMWH is a viable and preferred option. The use of oral anticoagulants, such as direct thrombin inhibitors, has been described in adult practice and may be a possibility for children in the future (12).

# VENOUS THROMBOEMBOLIC DISEASE ASSOCIATED WITH VMs

Due to the tortuous nature of the veins in the malformation and, in many cases, to their anatomical position, VMs may also pose a significant risk for venous thromboembolism (VTE) for many children and young adults. In addition to the small thromboses leading to painful phleboliths and DIC, deep vein thromboses are also well described in this cohort and are associated with morbidity and mortality (13).

Risk of VTE for the entire population increases with age, but children with VMs may have multiple additional risk factors specific to their VM: abnormal flow in abnormal vessels, episodes of inflammatory thrombophlebitis, relatively reduced mobility, and surgical interventions, including infections following procedures. They are also subject to the acquired risk factors that can affect other children and young adults: dehydration, trauma, use of the combined oral contraceptive pill, or pregnancy.

In younger children, the risk of VTE is relatively low, even for patients with VMs, but recognition of and counselling for VTE in the second decade is important for this group. Signs and symptoms of

Haematology

22

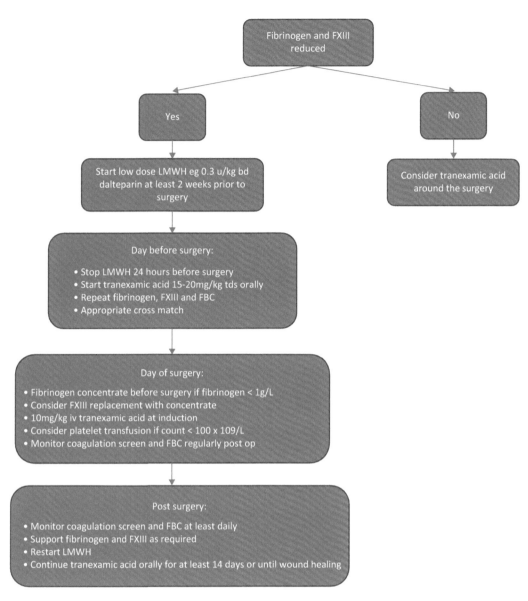

FIGURE 3.7 Flow chart of haematological management around surgery. LMWH: low molecular weight heparin, FBC: full blood count.

VTE are relatively poorly recognised in paediatric practice, and if the patient and family are not able to self-advocate, it can lead to delays in diagnosis and treatment. Times when thromboprophylaxis should be considered include:

- Situations leading to prolonged immobility
- Around the time of surgery
- If significant dehydration occurs
- Any other situation associated with infection or inflammation
- During pregnancy

Advice about lifestyle should include avoidance of smoking and maintaining a normal body mass index (BMI). Use of a combined oral contraceptive pill should generally be avoided given the well-recognised risk of VTE associated with these preparations in the general population. Given the small numbers involved, it is unlikely that this can be established as a specific risk in VM patients, but it seems a logical extrapolation to make, particularly in girls with large lower limb VMs. The risk for someone with a small lesion, not involving the lower limbs or pelvis, would be more debatable, and a sensible approach is to give individualised advice.

If a deep vein thrombosis or pulmonary embolism is diagnosed in a patient with a VM (or if it is suspected pending confirmatory imaging), anticoagulation with LMWH should be started with no delay (it should be noted that use of D dimer measurement as part of a diagnostic algorithm for VTE in this patient group is unhelpful because their baseline level is always elevated). For a child with DIC secondary to their VM, the LMWH dosing should be discussed with a centre experienced in managing such a clinical scenario, but if the baseline coagulation screen is normal, age and weight-based dosing can start.

The standard duration of anticoagulation for a precipitated VTE event would usually be 3 months for a DVT and 6 months for a pulmonary embolism. However, for children with VMs, the most significant risk factor is likely to be their VM, which is, therefore, life-long. Discussion with patients and their families about the risks and benefits of stopping anticoagulation is important. Until 2021, the only available oral anticoagulant was warfarin, with all its attendant difficulties (drug interactions, labile levels in association with illness, requirement for regular monitoring blood tests), making ongoing anticoagulation a significant challenge. Long-term treatment with LMWH is equally challenging for the majority of children and families. Rivaroxaban was the first direct oral anticoagulant (DOAC) to receive a paediatric licence for the treatment and prevention of venous thrombosis (after 5 days of treatment with LMWH). This has, therefore, provided an additional anticoagulation option for children with VTE associated with VMs and is likely to change the risk/benefit balance around ongoing anticoagulation in these patients. In some cases, a lower prophylaxis dose may be appropriate after an initial period of higher intensity treatment. It is hoped that other DOACs will become available in paediatric practice over the next few years.

In summary, active haematological expertise is a key part of the multidisciplinary team, especially for the most complex of cases both in terms of long-term management and during critical interventional radiology and surgical procedures to ensure the safety of the patient.

# REFERENCES

1. Redondo P, Aguado L, Marquina M, Paramo JA, Sierra A, Sánchez-Ibarrola A, Martínez-Cuesta A, Cabrera J, Angiogenic and prothrombotic markers in extensive slow-flow vascular malformations: Implications for antiangiogenic/antithrombotic strategies. *Br J Dermatol*. 2010 Feb 1;162(2):350–356. doi: 10.1111/j.1365-2133.2009.09513.x. Epub 2009 Sep 21. PMID: 19769632.
2. Levi M, Toh CH, Thachil J, Watson HG, Guidelines for the diagnosis and management of disseminated intravascular coagulation: British Committee for Standards in Haematology. *Br J Haematol*. 2009 Apr;145(1):24–33. doi: 10.1111/j.1365-2141.2009.07600.x. Epub 2009 Feb 12. PMID: 19222477
3. Mazoyer E, Enjolras O, Bisdorff A, Perdu J, Wassef M, Drouet L, Coagulation disorders in patients with venous malformation of the limbs and trunk: A case series of 118 patients. *Arch Dermatol*. 2008 Jul;144(7):861–867. doi: 10.1001/archderm.144.7.861. PMID: 18645137.
4. Dompmartin A, Acher A, Thibon P, Tourbach S, Hermans C, Deneys V, Pocock B, Lequerrec A, Labbé D, Barrellier MT, Vanwijck R, Vikkula M, Boon LM, Association of localized intravascular coagulopathy with venous malformations. *Arch Dermatol*. 2008 Jul;144(7):873–877. doi: 10.1001/archderm.144.7.873. PMID: 18645138; PMCID: PMC5572565.
5. New HV, Berryman J, Bolton-Maggs PHB, Cantwell C, Chalmers EA, Davies T, Gottstein R, Kelleher A, Kumar S, Morley SL, Stanworth, S.J. and (2016), Guidelines on transfusion for fetuses, neonates and older children. *Br J Haematol*. 2016 175: 784–828. https://doi.org/10.1111/bjh.14233
6. Zhuo KY, Russell S, Wargon O, Adams S, Localised intravascular coagulation complicating venous malformations in children: Associations and therapeutic options. *J Paediatr Child Health*. 2017 Aug;53(8):737–741. doi: 10.1111/jpc.13461. Epub 2017 Feb 7. PMID: 28169477
7. Aronniemi J, Långström S, Mattila KA, Mäkipernaa A, Salminen P, Pitkäranta A, Pekkola J, Lassila R, Venous malformations and blood coagulation in children. *Children (Basel)*. 2021 Apr 20;8(4):312. doi: 10.3390/children8040312. PMID: 33924092; PMCID: PMC8074292.
8. Fordham N, Clark J, Taylor A, Sibson K, Solman L, Glover M, Mathias M, Factor XIII levels correlate with fibrinogen concentrations in patients with venous malformations. *Haemophilia*. 2022 Nov;28(6):e251–e253. doi: 10.1111/hae.14654. Epub 2022 Sep 9. PMID: 36084282.
9. Mack JM, Verkamp B, Richter GT, Nicholas R, Stewart K, Crary SE, Effect of sirolimus on coagulopathy of slow-flow vascular malformations. *Pediatr Blood Cancer*. 2019 Oct;66(10):e27896. doi: 10.1002/pbc.27896. Epub 2019 Jun 28. PMID: 31250546.
10. Mazoyer E, Enjolras O, Laurian C, Houdart E, Drouet L, Coagulation abnormalities associated with extensive venous malformations of the limbs: Differentiation from Kasabach-Merritt syndrome. *Clin Lab Haematol*. 2002 Aug;24(4):243–251. doi: 10.1046/j.1365-2257.2002.00447.x. PMID: 12181029.
11. CRASH-2 trial collaborators, Shakur H, Roberts I, Bautista R, Caballero J, Coats T, Dewan Y, El-Sayed H, Gogichaishvili T, Gupta S, Herrera J, Hunt B, Iribhogbe P, Izurieta M, Khamis H, Komolafe E, Marrero MA, Mejía-Mantilla J, Miranda J, Morales C, Olaomi O, Olldashi F, Perel P, Peto R, Ramana PV, Ravi RR, Yutthakasemsunt S, Effects of tranexamic acid on death, vascular occlusive events, and blood transfusion in trauma patients with significant haemorrhage (CRASH-2): A randomised, placebo-controlled trial. *Lancet*. 2010 Jul 3;376(9734):23–32. doi: 1016/S0140-6736(10)60835-5. Epub 2010 Jun 14. PMID: 2055431911
12. Binet Q, Lambert C, Hermans C, Dabigatran etexilate in the treatment of localized intravascular coagulopathy associated with venous malformations. *Thromb Res*. 2018 Aug;168:114–120. doi: 10.1016/j.thromres.2018.06.013. Epub 2018 Jun 18. PMID: 30064682.
13. Mazereeuw-Hautier J, Syed S, Leisner RI, Harper JI, Extensive venous/lymphatic malformations causing life-threatening haematological complications. *Br J Dermatol*. 2007 Sep;157(3):558–563. doi: 10.1111/j.1365-2133.2007.08003.x. Epub 2007 Jun 15. PMID: 17573883.

Haematology

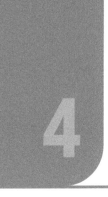

# 4  Psychology

Kristina Soon

## INTRODUCTION

The interplay between physical and psychological health is important to consider if the best patient-centred outcomes are to be achieved in paediatric settings. The physical challenges of living with a vascular malformation will affect the patient's psychological health, and psychological factors will affect the patient's experience of their physical health. How the patient's family and social network supports the developing child will also have a significant impact on physical and psychological outcomes.

A recent systematic review found that children with isolated vascular malformations showed comparable quality of life scores to children with mild urticaria or acne. Children with syndromic vascular malformations were found to have far lower quality of life scores, although the reviewers pointed out that research in children is very limited (1). Indeed, the studies included in this comprehensive review were small scale and utilised quality of life measures rather than robust mental health measures. Research in adults with vascular malformations shows reduced health-related quality of life as well as a more consistent pattern of increased psychological difficulties, especially in adults with syndromic vascular malformations (2). Childhood experiences and developmental opportunities are significant contributors to mental health in adulthood. As such, while children with vascular malformations may not show higher rates of frank mental health disorders, providing care that encompasses the psychological wellbeing of children can have not only an impact on their current quality of life but also set in motion important developmental trajectories that may reduce their likelihood of mental health problems in adulthood.

In the absence of research specific to paediatric vascular malformations, relevant findings from studies with related paediatric populations are below:

- A small number of studies have consistently shown that severity and size of visible difference is not associated with degree of psychological difficulties (3). The findings are mixed as to whether differences easily visible to others, e.g., on the face, are associated with poorer mental health than less visible differences, e.g., on the torso (4).
- There is a developing body of research that suggests that medical complexity, rather than appearance difference, especially the presence of chronic pain, can increase the likelihood of mental health difficulties in the patient (5, 6).
- Parental mental health and adjustment to the diagnosis of a chronic medical condition in their child is likely to significantly influence the psychological development of the child. As such, the psychological needs of the parent should also be considered when caring for a child patient (7).

Complex medical needs and procedures in the early years can result in increased risk of insecure attachment patterns between parent and child. However, follow-up studies have shown that attachment style will more likely be secure when stability returns to the child's and parent's lives (8). When the medical condition causes ongoing challenges, a sustained skew toward attachment insecurity has been observed (9). Whilst not problematic in itself, attachment insecurity is associated with a broad range of developmental and psychological difficulties in child- and adulthood.

DOI: 10.1201/9781003257417-4

Introduction

# COMMON PSYCHOLOGICAL CHALLENGES BY DEVELOPMENTAL STAGES

Psychological difficulties are typically the result of a complex interaction of biological, psychological, and social factors. As such, having a vascular malformation will not result in the same psychological outcomes for each young person. The following are the most common psychological challenges that present at different developmental stages. However, these will not apply to all patients in the same way, as each child and their family will bring with them a complex set of variables that will interact with the nature of the vascular malformation to influence the psychological impact of having a vascular malformation.

## INFANCY AND EARLY CHILDHOOD

Having a new healthy baby is a known stressor that can precipitate a range of stress-related reactions in parents, including major mental health difficulties. When a child has physical health differences, the stress can increase as a result of uncertainty about the infant's health and development and the extra health care burden of hospital attendances and daily management at home.

### Diagnosis

First, it should be acknowledged that many vascular malformations are not diagnosed until the child is beyond early childhood. The challenge of the discovery process for parents of infants has similarities to parents of older children, but there will be important differences, in particular, the impact of diagnosis on the child. The focus of this section is on diagnosis in infancy.

The direct psychological impact will be experienced by the parents/guardians and other family members and loved ones. The infant is unlikely to be aware or have any understanding of their physical health difference but will experience a secondary impact via the way in which the diagnosis and related experiences affect their carers as well as the way their carers interact with them and allow them to interact with the world around them. As such, a key role for health care professionals at this developmental stage will be in ensuring that the experience of the vascular malformation and the care around it does not impair normative parenting behaviours. This is important in ensuring the child's best start to an adaptive psychological and developmental trajectory.

### Grief, Loss, and Sadness

Immediate reactions are often characterised by shock, difficulty in grasping information, and a desire to regain some sense of control over child and family life, which can be why, for many parents, there is a sense of relief when a diagnosis is made. However, following shortly after the period of high stress, there can be a period of bereavement. While many family allies and health care professionals can be surprised by the parents' feelings of sadness and loss, especially if the child is otherwise physically well or has a good prognosis, bereavement is an important process by which the parents let go of previously held hopes and expectations for the birth and imagined life of their child and an adjustment to a more realistic set of expectations given the specific needs of their child. Many parents can feel confused about their intense sadness, whilst cradling their baby who is fundamentally healthy, and feel guilty, often comparing their situation to other parents whose children are much more impaired.

---

**CASE EXAMPLE**

One parent had experienced a difficult childhood themselves, including peer victimisation and loneliness throughout school. They had dreamt of giving their own child a more carefree upbringing than their own that would help their child to develop the self-confidence the parent had always yearned for. Finding out that their child would have a visible difference as a result of the vascular malformation plunged this parent into a deep sadness and despair that they would not be able to give their child the life that they had hoped – that they would not be able to protect their own child from the pain that they had suffered in childhood.

---

## Managing Medical and Daily Care

Supporting parents to develop good skills, knowledge, and confidence in delivering daily care will help to improve the condition of the vascular malformation as well as set up a good framework for future management as the child becomes older. Taking time at this early stage to ensure that the parents have good information and confidence in providing care to their child is contingent on a trusting relationship between the health care team and the family. Establishing epistemic trust at this early stage will help parents, and, later on, the child, accept the advice and guidance of the health care team.

Delivering care to small children is sometimes viewed as easier, in that they are less able to dissent than an older child. However, small children can become extremely distressed when experiencing pain and discomfort whilst not being able to understand why. Additionally, inflicting distress and discomfort on their own child, even for the "right" reasons, can be extremely distressing to the parent. It can be difficult to encourage the child to collaborate with parents and health care professionals when they can't understand the purpose of the procedures due to their early cognitive and language processing ability.

Whilst it can be tempting to use physical size and strength as the means of ensuring that the small child receives the care that they require, this kind of control can contribute to a pattern of aversive and adversarial interactions between parents, health care professionals, and the child, which can be difficult to reverse as the child gets older. As such, even though the child is still small, it is important to support the establishment of positive and collaborative behaviours at home and in health care settings. These include:

- Setting up a calming environment for care, e.g., low lights, quietness, relaxing music, carers modelling a calm and quiet demeanour.
- Explaining to a verbal child, in language that they can understand, what is going to happen and why. Predictability reduces pain perception as well as anxiety (10). It also establishes trust between the child and the adult carers.
- Utilising strategies for reducing distress such as medical pain control, deep breathing, gentle massage, or distraction can help to reduce distress in the moment as well as help to develop a toolkit of effective coping strategies for the future. Finding the best strategies for each child and family may take some experimentation. This can be a collaborative experience of discovery for the child and carers that further develops trust and cooperation.
- Any patient, regardless of age, can feel a sense of loss of control over their bodies and their lives. Helping even the youngest patients feel that they have some control can reduce pain and distress from procedures as well as develop a pattern of collaboration between the child and adult carers. Examples of giving the child control include encouraging them to select which favourite toy to bring or television show to watch, which part of their body they want to focus on first or being encouraged to participate, e.g., by handing the parent a dressing or choosing and adhering a plaster.
- In the midst of multiple additional challenges to parents and health care professionals, it can be easy to forget how hard it can be for a young child to have to experience a vascular malformation and the care related to it. Not acknowledging these extra demands on the child can result in resentment and hopelessness, which can lead to treatment difficulties in the future. Remembering to praise the child and to establish a simple reward system for each time the child manages yet another treatment or hospital visit can help to develop a sense of mastery as well as trust in the adult carers.

## Sharing the News

A recent paper on the psychosocial impact of vascular malformations on children and families named one of the key challenges of this early period of adjustment as informing family and friends of the vascular malformation and taking the child who has a visible difference to public places (11).

While still adjusting to their child's vascular malformation themselves, parents can feel anxious and uncertain about who to tell about the vascular malformation and how much to tell. Parents can be concerned about causing distress to others or may worry about the reaction, such as being pitied or stigmatised. Taking their new baby to public places can also be a source of anxiety with parents feeling fearful about the reactions of others to their child's appearance. However, being able to speak openly about the vascular malformation not only sets a good example for the child as they grow up but also can open up opportunities for the parents to seek support and comfort from the people around them. Open communication between parent, health care professionals and child will also facilitate good collaborative management of the vascular malformation going forward.

There is now a sizeable research base underpinning good practice in supporting the disclosure of medical conditions (12), which emphasises the role of the health care team in supporting or obstructing this process. Health care teams can support disclosure by providing parents with clear information using vocabulary that the parent can understand and then use themselves. Supporting parents to be able to express "not knowing" will also be important as the range of questions parents face is unlimited and the fear of being unable to answer a question can feel overwhelming. Parents can also be supported in sharing their child's condition in a graded fashion by identifying the people who they expect will respond better to the news or who need to know and to "practice" sharing the information with them first before moving onto people they feel more worried about telling.

Parents of children with visible medical conditions often experience challenges from strangers as well as loved ones such as staring, intrusive questions, or unsolicited advice. A vascular malformation that has the appearance of a bruise or swelling can also cause alarm in others that the child is being abused. Expressing sympathy and normalising this experience to parents can be validating. Encouraging parents to rehearse how they would like to respond to these kinds of situations can help to prepare them for the real experience and to avoid feeling paralysed in the moment.

As the child becomes verbal and starts to spend more time amongst others, such as at nursery or a playground, the child will also be faced with stares, questions, and comments like their parents. To support the child to feel confident in responding to these, it is important for parents to model desirable behaviours while the child is still very young, even pre-verbal, so that these are the actions that the child internalises and then naturally adopts as they get older. Speaking openly within the family and to strangers and in a calm and contained way will show the child that talking about the vascular malformation is not a problem. Choosing vocabulary that is developmentally appropriate will give them the best chance for learning useful words to describe their vascular malformation to others when the time comes. For example, vascular malformation is quite a mouthful and not easily understandable to others. Terms such as "birthmark" or "squiggly veins", whilst not strictly accurate, can be easier terms for children to use and for others to understand.

---

## TOP TIPS FOR HEALTH CARE PROFESSIONALS: EARLY CHILDHOOD

- Don't try to rationalise parents out of their sadness. It needs to run its course, during which time, sympathy and patience is the best help.

- Provide as much information as you can to help parents to adjust to the VM, but do not feel pressured to provide information that you don't have. It is difficult to tolerate uncertainty, but this is an inevitability of parenting a child with additional needs.

- Encourage parents and professional carers to establish collaborative strategies for medical procedures and daily care to develop trust and cooperation between adults and child rather than relying on force and coercion.

- Encourage parents to speak openly about the VM with their child from an early age so that the child learns useful words and information as well as learning that talking about their vascular malformation is fine.

---

## PRESCHOOL AND PRIMARY SCHOOL

As children start to develop a clearer sense of themselves as separate entities to their parents, and as their physical, cognitive, and verbal development progresses, their experience and understanding of their vascular malformation become more complex. The main developmental tasks during this age range are to learn how to independently relate to peers and adults beyond their immediate family. This is also the time when children rapidly develop a broad range of skills including school subjects, play activities, sports, and hobbies, as well as activities of daily living such as managing personal hygiene, and organising their time and space such as tidying their rooms, getting dressed for school on time, and preparing foods and drinks. Success or failure in developing these skills can affect the child's sense of self and their confidence in their own agency. This is also the time when social skills need to develop rapidly in order for the child to be able to engage, increasingly independently, with the world around them.

### Developing a Sense of Self in Relation to Others

Children will tend to start noticing appearance differences between people, such as hair and skin colour and body size, and may start asking questions about their vascular malformation around the age of 4 when they realise, for example, that their parent or sibling does not have a vascular malformation also. The social meaning of looking different, such as of being "less than", is noticeably absent in these early stages, giving parents and carers a window of opportunity to ensure that the child receives positive messages about appearance differences. Similarly, their peers may notice the vascular malformation in a curious way. As children get older and reach an age at which social comparison becomes increasingly important in primary school, a child with a vascular malformation is likely to start receiving negative messages about themselves about looking different, being less able in sport or requiring assistance at or being frequently absent from school. The child will also notice themselves that they may be lagging behind their peers in some way. As such, even in the absence of explicit negative messages from others, a child can still start to develop a sense of themselves as being not as good as their peers.

Parents and health care professionals alike, sensitised to the distress of the child, are sometimes tempted to minimise or hide the difference such as through camouflage make up or clothing. Whilst hiding the vascular malformation may provide short-term relief from stress, this can have the unintended effect of implicitly communicating to the child that their difference is shameful and should be hidden from sight.

If the vascular malformation is evident to others, whether that means the lesion itself is visible, its impact on the child's functioning is evident, or the care required is observable to others, it is almost inevitable that the child will experience comments, questions, or stares which can cause them to feel embarrassed, confused, or hurt. Although upsetting, the majority of these are not intended to be hurtful, but some may have the explicit malicious purpose of hurting the child's feelings. It will be important for the child to learn how to distinguish intention so that they understand the different reasons why others may behave in a hurtful way and to help them to formulate how best to respond in the moment. Even when faced with an innocent question about their vascular malformation, children can feel upset, unprepared and socially awkward, resulting in the young person feeling even more negative about themselves.

Social support and a good social network are known to be psychologically protective to all children and adults. Because making friends can be difficult when a child has a physical difference, extra support and encouragement in developing good social skills and a supportive social network from a young age will be protective as the child experiences challenges such as bullying and transition to secondary school.

The quotes below are taken from a study with 11–14-year-old children with visible differences, including vascular malformations (13), and provide examples of the social and emotional challenges that children can face.

*"I don't get invited to people's birthday parties and … I invite them but they don't invite me."*

**(P1)**

*"When I am feeling upset, it's just like the words they say keep going around in my head. Stuff like you are ugly, you are ugly, keeps going 'round in my head."*

**(P8)**

*"I usually went up to my room and said I was fine and just felt bad. And then the next day like put on a face like a mask of how I am fine but I'm not really."*

**(P2)**

The building blocks for managing the impact of stigmatising social experiences should begin early in the child's life.

- Families should be encouraged to speak openly with their child about their vascular malformation and with the people around them. Even when still pre-verbal, children will be noticing and copying their parent's actions and emotions. Parents who avoid talking about the vascular malformation may inadvertently convey a sense of stigma about the vascular malformation.
- Whilst it can feel extremely intrusive and tiresome to parents to have to respond to questions and comments from family, friends, and strangers about the vascular malformation, modelling openness to discussing the vascular malformation with others, within reason, can normalise the experience as well as demonstrate to the child how to answer questions and what to say. Reacting angrily to questions, avoiding public places, or concealing their child's difference may inadvertently convey to their child that their vascular malformation is problematic.
- Modelling positive behaviours should be accompanied by explicit support. These include developing an age-appropriate vocabulary, encouraging their child to speak about the vascular malformation, first within the family and then broadening to other social contexts as they become more confident, providing their child with opportunities to explain their experience of the vascular malformation to others in response to their questions. For children who feel anxious about speaking to adults or peers, it may be helpful to do some practice at home in a light-hearted way. In this way, when the young person is faced with questions or stares, they know exactly what to do and they can feel confident in their response.

- Distinguishing between honest, albeit insensitive, curiosity and malicious acts can help the child to understand how best to respond. Understanding that the other person is only interested or concerned for them can lead to a friendly and informative conversation about the vascular malformation. The visible difference charity Changing Faces coined the 'Explain, Reassure, Divert' technique, for example. On the other hand, interactions that are meant to hurt the young person should be named as such and reported to someone who can give a clear message to the perpetrator that the behaviour was unacceptable. Support might also need to be provided to the child to prevent them from internalising the negative message that they have experienced. Distinguishing intent can result in not only more effective reactions but also help the child to understand that the world is not a bad place and that people, while sometimes ignorant about vascular malformation and insensitive, are also not all bad.
- It is helpful to encourage parents to discuss their child's vascular malformation-related needs ahead of the start of school. This way the school can be clear about the nature of the vascular malformation and the care required as well as being clear about how the parents would like daily care and social difficulties to be handled by the school. Consistency across home and school will set clear expectations and boundaries that will help the child feel safer and more confident.
- It can be very upsetting to parents to hear that their child has been hurt by someone because of their VM. This can trigger reactions in the parent that might not be helpful to the child, such as angrily confronting the other child or their parents or taking the child out of school. Sometimes the best role for the parent is to simply validate the child's distress and help to soothe them in the best way that they know. Using the experience as a way of understanding their child's world and learning how to deal collaboratively with challenges better in the future is also important. Solutions from parents may not always feel helpful to the child and vice versa. Shared problem solving is usually the best way of coming up with a mutually acceptable plan of action.

---

## TOP TIPS FOR HEALTH CARE PROFESSIONALS: PRIMARY SCHOOL

Support parents to scaffold good social skills development in their child by modelling prosocial behaviours, encouraging opportunities for social interactions, and developing strong, supportive social networks around their child.

Normalise the experience of feeling hurt by questions, comments, and stares. Encourage parents to work together with their child to understand the intentions behind the behaviours of others in order to work out how best to respond.

Encourage parents to support their child in engaging in as many developmentally appropriate opportunities that they can in order to facilitate their cognitive, physical, social, and emotional development alongside their peers. Developing confidence in other areas of life will help the child to build a positive and multi-faceted sense of themselves.

Support parents to establish good relationships with their health care network, families, friends, and educators. This not only models good social skills and positive help-seeking for their child, but it will also help to ensure that the child is well supported as they become increasingly independent from their family.

---

## ADOLESCENCE

Adolescence is well-known as a time of intense physical, emotional, and social development. This is often a challenging time for young people and their parents regardless of health status. Adolescents typically start to seek the independence of adulthood yet lack the cognitive development and life experience to be as effective as they and their parents would like. There is a tension between desire for independence from family and anxiety about rejection by peers. Social rejection for "being different" and disagreements and frustrations about managing the condition can result in conflict and withdrawal between family members and despair and humiliation for the young person.

The major developmental tasks at this stage relate to developing a sense of self in relation to their peers and the world around them, e.g., values, behaviours, and friendship groups as well as preparing for adulthood such as through deciding on a career path and envisioning the kind of future that is consistent with newly developing values, e.g., getting married and having children, planning a fulfilling career, travelling or having their own home.

## Identity

Defining one's own identity is a challenge faced by most adolescents. This can be a painful and confusing process for all. Vascular malformations can add further complication if the vascular malformation and its corollary of medical/daily care, limitations to daily activities, and influence on the young person's sense of self as different or defective obscure other aspects of the young person's sense of self. The identity of being "sick" or "different" can come to dominate a young person's sense of who they are. It can become difficult for the young person and the people around them to notice other, equally important aspects of themselves such as being smart, conscientious, funny, kind, artistic, impatient, athletic, etc.

Young people who feel marginalised and different can also struggle with the prospect of forming intimate relationships. Anxiety-provoking for most adolescents, low self-esteem, feeling unattractive, social isolation, or feeling worried about their intimate partner discovering a hidden difference can cause this important development milestone to feel out of reach, resulting in a sense of alienation, hopelessness, and despair. Furthermore, it can be difficult for many young people to share these types of worries with their parents, which contributes further to a sense of hopelessness. Establishing relationships with others who the young person can talk to about their worries can be the best way that parents can support their child through this difficult stage. Sources of help can come from favourite family members, peer networks, school counsellors, trusted health care professionals, or mental health professionals.

## Planning for the Future

A great deal of time in adolescence is spent trying to envisage possible futures, often trying on different roles and personas as a means of working out what fits best. A young person with a vascular malformation may struggle to look forward to their future without help in understanding how their vascular malformation will affect them and how it may influence their ability to achieve desired goals. The absence of hope for the future can result in demotivation and despair in the young person as well as alienation and resentment in relation to their peers who are already planning for their futures.

Parents may also feel concerned about building their child's hopes and aspirations if they turn out to be unrealistic. If the young person has continuing medical needs, conversations between parent and child may still be dominated by the vascular malformation and vascular malformation-related care, which obstructs the opportunities to discuss hopes and plans for the future.

---

### CASE EXAMPLE

A 15-year-old girl had a vascular malformation affecting the length of one leg, which grew as she reached adolescence, resulting in a noticeable difference in length between her two legs. As a result, she was no longer able to compete at an elite level in her chosen sport. This young woman had committed most of her time and energy since early primary school to achieving international sporting success and had started to realise that she could no longer perform at an elite level due to her leg length discrepancy. She was referred to psychology feeling depressed and anxious. Her parents expressed frustration that their child had withdrawn from them and felt unable to help her. With encouragement, the young woman explained that she felt like a failure in her sport, yet felt she had no other options in life, leaving her with a bleak future. Allowing her to grieve for the loss of her hopes for a future in sport and supporting her to notice the many other talents and strengths that she possessed resulted in the young woman being able to envisage an alternative and satisfying future for herself outside of her sport. She began spending (and enjoying) more time with her friends and re-focused her attention and motivation toward academic study, which resulted in a significant rapid improvement in her grades which she hoped would allow her to study law at university. With help, this young woman was able to realise how much more there was to the person she thought she was and how she could be happy, fulfilled, and successful.

---

## Treatment Adherence

Brief mention should be made of treatment adherence and adolescent patients. The literature is very clear that treatment adherence tends to deteriorate during the adolescent period across a range of different medical conditions. The negotiation of increasing behavioural independence from parents, the ongoing development of cognitive function, especially in executive functions, the extraordinary physiological strain of physical development, and the acute anxiety about social belongingness all contribute to great difficulty in maintaining good treatment adherence for both parents and patient. Ensuring that the young person is included in major treatment decisions and feels that they have some control over the treatment process will be helpful in maximising the chances of success. However, it will also be important to be able to tolerate some deterioration in treatment adherence and the subsequent impact on symptoms. A health care professional can be key to working out which aspects of care are non-negotiable and where there can be some flexibility and tolerance in order to maintain good relationships between adolescent, parents, and health care team.

---

## TOP TIPS FOR HEALTH CARE PROFESSIONALS: ADOLESCENTS

From as early as possible, try to involve the young person in the consultation – directing questions about symptoms at them rather than just their parent and asking for the young person's opinion when considering treatment options.

Accept that the young person will want to do things their way, even if it means a deterioration in symptom care. Allow them control in some areas but be clear about what is non-negotiable.

Check that the young person has started considering plans and goals for the future.

Suggest positive role models that the young person can relate to on social media or through service-user networks and peer support.

---

## THE ROLE OF THE PSYCHOLOGIST

It is important to remember that, when faced with a medical condition or difficult information, distress, disagreement, and resistance are all typical reactions. To refer a patient or their parent who is expressing these feelings in response to life-changing information to a mental health professional can feel deeply invalidating. Normative reactions to difficult news should be allowed to resolve naturally.

However, reactions from parent or child that may appear to be typical, initially, can persist or worsen to the point that they are obstructing important processes, such as the parent–child relationship, the child's development, or optimal medical care. It is at this point that a referral to a specialist mental health professional may be indicated.

There are also particular areas of care relating to the vascular malformation that can feel beyond the capabilities of most parents for which a psychologist can be of help. These are typically pain management, entrenched treatment adherence difficulties, procedural fear and appearance-related difficulties, such as persistent peer victimisation or poor self-image and mood disorders in adolescence. The psychologist is a key member of the vascular malformation multidisciplinary team and plays an important role in achieving the best result for the patient.

## REFERENCES

1. Nguyen, H, Bonadurer, G, Tollefson, M (2018) Vascular malformations and health-related quality of life: A systematic review and meta-analysis. *JAMA Dermatology*, Vol 154, Issue 6, 661–669.
2. Pang, C, Gibson, M, Nisbet, R, Evans, N, Khalifa, M, Papadopoulou, A, Tsui, J, Hamilton, G, Brookes, J, Lim, CS (2022) Quality of life and mental health of patients with vascular malformations in a single specialist center in the United Kingdom. *Journal of Vascular Surgery: Venous and Lymphatic Disorders*, Vol 10, Issue 1, 159–169.
3. Rumsey, N, Harcourt, D (2007) Visible difference amongst children and adolescents: Issues and interventions. *Developmental Neurorehabilitation*, Vol 10, Issue 2, 113–123.
4. Ambrose, J (2020) The impact of stigma and visible difference on children and adolescents living with physical health conditions (Doctoral Dissertation) London: UCL.
5. Oduber, CE, Khemlani, K, Sillevis Smitt, JH, Hennekam, RC, van der Horst, CM (2010) Baseline quality of life in patients with Klippel-Trenaunay syndrome. *Journal of Plastic, Reconstructive & Aesthetic Surgery*, Vol 63, Issue 4, 603–609.
6. Soon, K, Mason, R, Martinez, AE, & Mellerio, JE (2020) The psychological functioning of children with Epidermolysis Bullosa (EB) and its relationship with specific aspects of disease. *British Journal of Dermatology* doi:10.1111/bjd.18592
7. Sawyer, M, Streiner, D, Antoniou, G, Toogood, I, Rice, M (1998) Influence of parental and family adjustment on the later psychological adjustment of children treated for cancer. *Journal of the American Academy of Child and Adolescent Psychiatry*, Vol 37, Issue 8, Aug, 815–822.

Psychology

8. Maris, C, Endriga, M, Speltz, M, Jones, K, DeKlyen, M (2000) Are infants with Oro-facial clefts at risk for insecure mother-child attachments? *Cleft Lip and Palate Journal*, Vol 37, Issue 3, 257–265.

9. Soon, K (2016) Towards and explanatory model of psychological functioning in children and adolescents with congenital dermatological disfigurement (Doctoral Dissertation) London: UCL.

10. Oka, K, Chapman, C, Barkhwa, K, Shimizu, O, Noma, N, Takeichi, O, Imamura, Y, Oi, Y (2010) Predictability of painful stimulation modulates subjective and physiological responses. *Journal of Pain*, Vol 11, Issue 3 (March) 239–246.

11. Espinel, A Bauman, N (2018) Psychosocial impact of vascular anomalies on children and their families. *Otolaryngologic Clinics of North America*, Vol 51, 99–110.

12. Evangeli, M & Kagee, A (2016) A model of caregiver paediatric HIV disclosure decision-making. *Psychology, Health & Medicine*, Vol 21, Issue 3, 338–353.

13. Beak, S (2014) Social rejection in adolescents with visible facial disfigurement: A qualitative study (Doctoral Dissertation) London: UCL.

# Infantile Haemangiomas 5

Lea Solman

## INTRODUCTION

Infantile haemangiomas (IHs) are the most common vascular tumours of childhood, affecting 4–5% of infants (1). They are more common in premature or low birth-weight infants, females, and Caucasians. Risk factors also include increased maternal age, multiple pregnancies, preeclampsia, family history of IH, and placental anomalies such as placenta previa, placental abruption, and abnormal insertion of the umbilical cord (1). IHs arise in the first weeks of life, then grow rapidly for the first few months (2). Precursor lesions can be present at birth or appear early in the neonatal period, usually occurring as an area of pallor due to local vasoconstriction or as telangiectatic macules. IHs usually complete their growth at 5 months of age, although the proliferative phase may continue until around 12 months of age (3). Regression is complete in 90% of cases by the age of 4 years, although for deeper lesions, it may be slower and continue until the age of 7 or 8 years (4). After regression, up to 70% of IHs leave behind residual skin changes (19).

The aetiology of IHs is still poorly understood. A leading hypothesis is that circulating endothelial progenitor cells migrate to locations in which conditions such as hypoxia and developmental field disturbances are favourable for growth (5). The majority of IHs do not require treatment, but about 15% of all IH result in complications, such as obstruction of the visual axis or airway, ulceration, or disfigurement, necessitating therapeutic intervention.

## CLINICAL FEATURES

The majority of haemangiomas are solitary, but multiple lesions occur in up to 20% of patients (6). They have a predilection for the head and neck but can appear anywhere on the skin, mucosa, or, rarely, internal organs. Based on their depth during the proliferative phase, they can be classified into superficial, deep, mixed, or arrested/minimal growth IHs. Superficial IHs (Figure 5.1) are located in the upper dermis, appear as bright red vascular plaques or nodules, and are the most common type. Deep IHs (Figure 5.2) extend to adipose tissue and usually present as a subcutaneous, compressible, bluish vascular nodule with or without a central telangiectatic patch. They may not be noted until the infant is 3–4 months of age and can be mistaken for venous or lymphatic malformations. Mixed IHs (Figure 5.3) have both superficial and deep components. Arrested/minimal growth IHs show very little proliferation and present as a fine or coarse telangiectatic patch (Figure 5.4). In about a third of arrested/minimal growth IHs, proliferation is present, usually as small papules at the periphery (7), which are a useful diagnostic clue. The majority of arrested/minimal growth IHs occur on the lower body and also show a tendency toward acral locations (7). They can be often mistaken for capillary malformations. In the past, superficial IHs have been called "capillary" or "strawberry" haemangiomas, and deep IHs were named "cavernous" haemangiomas. These terms are now obsolete and should be avoided.

Based on their morphology, IHs can be divided into localised, segmental, indeterminate, or multifocal. Localised IHs are spatially confined, often surrounding a central focal point (Figure 5.5a,b),

DOI: 10.1201/9781003257417-5

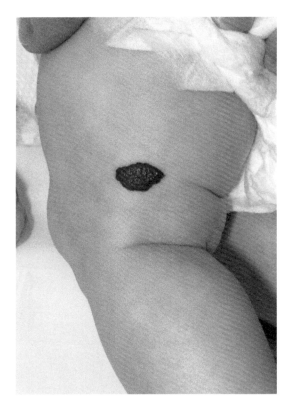

FIGURE 5.1 Superficial IH of the left lateral thigh in a 13-week-old female.

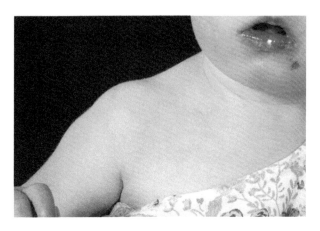

FIGURE 5.2 Deep IH of the right upper chest wall with prominent draining veins in a 1-year-old female.

whereas segmental IHs involve an anatomic territory, with many corresponding to known embryologic developmental units (8) (Figure 5.6). Indeterminate IHs lack the round or ovoid shape of many localised IHs yet are smaller in size than classic segmental lesions. Multifocal IHs are defined as five or more IH lesions, and in most children, these are limited to the skin. Visceral IHs, apart from liver IHs, are rare.

## ASSOCIATED DEVELOPMENTAL ANOMALIES

A small subset of children with IHs in certain locations can present with developmental abnormalities. Infants with a segmental/large haemangioma of the face, neck, and/or scalp should be evaluated for

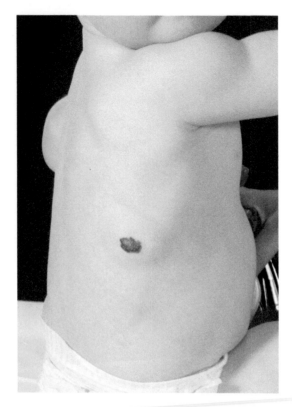

FIGURE 5.3 Mixed IH of the right mid-back in a 10-month-old male.

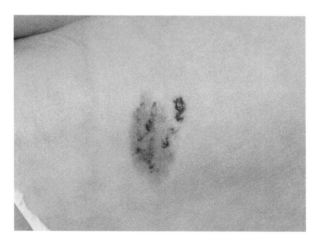

FIGURE 5.4 Minimal (arrested growth) infantile haemangioma of the left anterior thigh in a 7-month-old male.

PHACE syndrome (**p**osterior fossa anomalies, **h**aemangioma, **a**rterial anomalies, **c**ardiac anomalies, and **e**ye anomalies). The acronym PHACE(S) is sometimes used in the presence of ventral developmental defects, such as a sternal cleft and/or a supraumbilical raphe. Congenital abnormalities of the medium size arteries of the head and neck are the most frequent extracutaneous anomaly in PHACE, occurring in approximately 40% of patients (9, 10), including dysplasia, narrowing, or aberrant vessel course (11). Children with PHACE syndrome are at risk of progressive narrowing of the cerebral arteries, thus, increasing the risk of acute ischaemic stroke. Structural brain anomalies occur in 41% of patients, most commonly unilateral cerebral hypoplasia, Dandy–Walker variants, and true Dandy–Walker malformation (11). In a study from an international PHACE registry, 41% of patients were found to have a cardiac anomaly, most commonly an aberrant subclavian artery, coarctation of the aorta, or ventricular septal

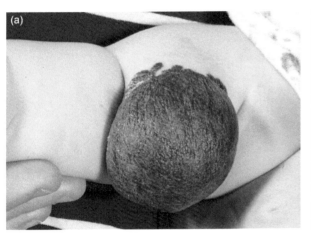
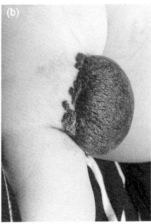

FIGURE 5.5 Localised IH of the right medial upper arm in a 7-month-old girl shown from the front (a) and side (b).

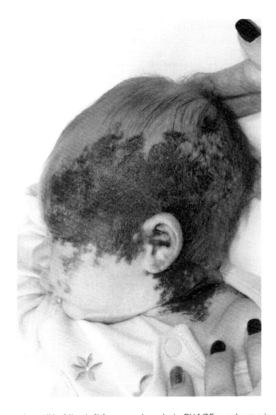

FIGURE 5.6 Segmental plaque type IH of the left face and scalp in PHACE syndrome in a 1-month-old female.

defect (10). Ocular abnormalities occur in 16% of patients (12). Patients with PHACE syndrome are also at risk of neurodevelopmental changes, speech and language delay, endocrine abnormalities, headaches, hearing loss, and dental issues.

IHs located over the lumbosacral spine (Figure 5.7) can be associated with underlying regional developmental abnormalities. Various acronyms for this condition have been described during the years: SACRAL (13) (spinal dysraphism, anogenital, cutaneous, renal and urologic anomalies, angioma of lumbosacral localisation), PELVIS (14) (perineal haemangioma, external genitalia malformations, lipomyelomeningocele, vesicorenal abnormalities, imperforate anus, and skin tag), and LUMBAR (15) (lower body IH, urogenital anomalies and ulceration, myelopathy, bone deformities, anorectal malformations, arterial anomalies, and renal anomalies). IHs that are adjacent to but do not cross the midline

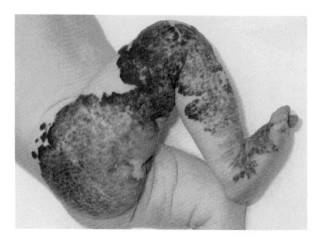

FIGURE 5.7 Segmental plaque type IH of the right lateral leg and buttock in LUMBAR syndrome in a 2-month-old female.

usually do not warrant further investigation (16). Segmental IHs of the gluteal cleft and lumbosacral spine extending over the midline are the greatest concern and should be investigated.

# DIAGNOSIS AND INVESTIGATIONS

IHs are usually diagnosed clinically. Imaging investigations such as Doppler ultrasound or magnetic resonance imaging (MRI) are required if the diagnosis is unclear, usually to distinguish deep IH from another type of vascular anomaly. Biopsy of the lesion is rarely required and can usually be reserved for lesions with an unusual appearance and/or atypical features in the clinical history, especially if a malignant lesion is suspected.

The proliferative phase of IHs shows lobules and sheets of tightly packed, capillary-size vascular channels lined by plump, bland endothelial cells with thin basement membranes surrounded by pericytes (Figure 5.8). There is usually minimal intervening stroma, composed mainly of fibroblasts and other mononuclear cells. Mitoses may be present, especially in young children, but no atypical mitotic figures or anaplasia are present. The later involuting phase is represented by a reduced number of vascular channels, flattening of the endothelium, and increased interstitial fibrosis. The larger 'feeder vessels' (arteries and veins) appear relatively prominent, as the capillary component regresses. In involuted cases, identification of the lesion may be difficult, with only scattered abnormal capillaries remaining within a fibrofatty background, although the large feeding/draining vessels can remain.

It is suggested that the endothelial cells in proliferating IH are likely arrested in an early developmental stage of differentiation. The abnormal endothelial cells of IH express endothelial markers, such as

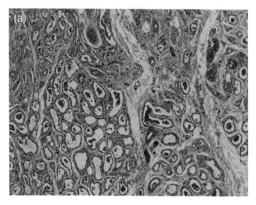
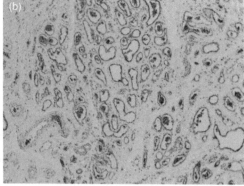

FIGURE 5.8 Photomicrographs of an IH. (a) H&E staining original magnification x100, (b) GLUT-1 staining original magnification x100, demonstrating skin with an underlying poorly circumscribed and unencapsulated lesion composed of numerous small capillary type vascular channels with no atypia. Characteristically, lesional endothelial cells strongly express GLUT-1.

Infantile Haemangiomas

CD31 and CD34, but characteristically express glucose transporter protein isoform 1 (GLUT1), which is normally expressed in placenta and perineurium. Smooth muscle actin (SMA) staining highlights pericytes and vascular smooth muscle (17).

In some IHs, additional investigations are required. In patients with segmental/large IH of the face, neck, and/or scalp, an MRI of the head and magnetic resonance angiography (MRA) of the head and neck is required to exclude posterior fossa anomalies and anomalies of cerebral arteries. These patients also require an echocardiogram (ECHO) and electrocardiogram (ECG) to exclude cardiac anomalies. They also need to be referred to an ophthalmology team to rule out eye anomalies. In patients with segmental IH of the gluteal cleft or lumbosacral spine, MRI of the whole spine with contrast should be performed to exclude spinal abnormalities, spinal haemangiomas, spinal dysraphism, or tethering of the spinal cord. They should also have an ultrasound of the abdomen to rule out renal/urological abnormalities. Finally, patients with liver IH can develop acquired hypothyroidism due to production of type 3 iodothyronine deiodinase. For that reason, thyroid function tests should be done in all patients with multiple liver haemangiomas (18). Patients with suspected airway haemangiomas should be referred to an ENT specialist.

# COMPLICATIONS

Most cutaneous IHs are not complicated and do not require intervention. During the proliferative phase, an IH may ulcerate or cause functional impairment. Up to 70% of IHs leave behind residual skin changes, including telangiectasia, fibrofatty tissue, redundant skin, atrophy, dyspigmentation, and scar, especially in lesions with a history of past ulceration (19).

Ulceration is the most common complication of an IH, occurring in about 16% of patients, usually before 4 months of age (20). It is more frequent in rapidly proliferating IHs and in areas of repeated trauma, pressure, and maceration (Figure 5.9). Large, superficial, and plaque IHs are more likely to ulcerate. Moisture and maceration seem to particularly promote ulceration; a prospective study showed that 50% of patients with an IH in the nappy area and 30% of patients with an IH on the lip developed an ulceration (20). Early grey or white discoloration of the IH surface in infants younger than 3 months might be an early sign of ulceration (20). Ulceration on the lip can cause difficulties feeding due to pain (Figure 5.10), and patients can develop faltering growth. Ulceration prevention measures are not well established, but liberal use of an emollient such as petroleum jelly and avoidance of friction/irritation is recommended. Treatment of ulceration is discussed below.

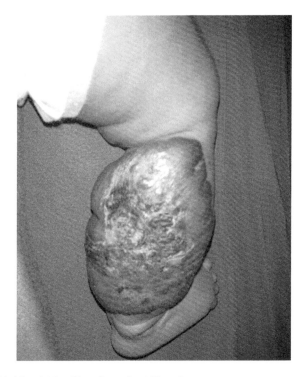

FIGURE 5.9 Ulcerated IH of the right calf in a 2-month-old female.

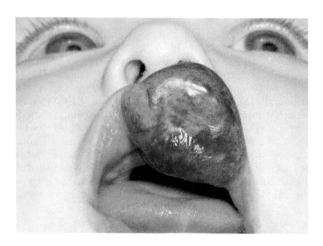

FIGURE 5.10 Ulcerated IH of the upper lip.

Bleeding is commonly feared by the parents or caregivers, but it is very rarely profuse and can be stopped by the application of direct pressure.

Peri-ocular IH can cause ptosis, strabismus, astigmatism, and, most importantly, amblyopia and visual impairment. Predictive factors for ocular complications in patients with peri-ocular IH are a diameter greater than 1 cm, a deep component, and upper eyelid involvement, with size being the most consistent predictor (21). These patients should be promptly referred to an ophthalmologist and treated with systemic beta-blockers.

Airway IHs can occur in children without cutaneous IHs; however, the risk of airway IHs is higher in patients with a segmental IH in a beard distribution (S3 cutaneous segment) especially in bilateral lesions (Figure 5.11). This distribution includes the preauricular skin, mandible, lower lip, chin, and/or

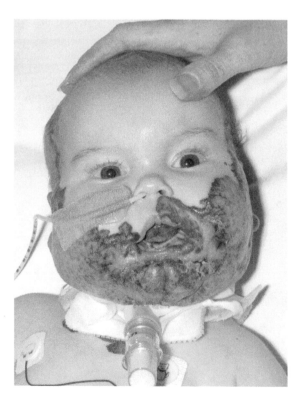

FIGURE 5.11 Segmental plaque type IH in beard distribution in a 5-month-old female.

Infantile Haemangiomas

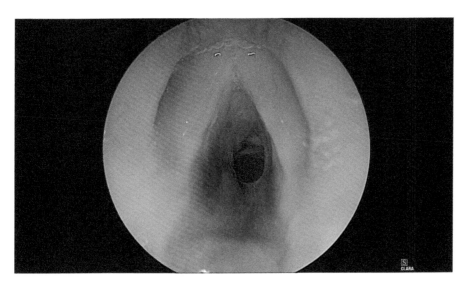

FIGURE 5.12 IH of the airway.

anterior neck (22). Airway IHs usually involve the subglottis, which is the narrowest part of the child's airway and are mostly located in its left posterolateral part (23) (Figure 5.12). Affected infants may develop stridor, hoarseness, and respiratory failure between 4 and 12 weeks of age due to rapid growth of the IH. Patients with suspected airway IHs need to be urgently discussed in a multidisciplinary setting, including the ENT team, ahead of endoscopic assessment and treatment.

In most children with multiple IHs (arbitrarily defined as ≥5 generally small, localised IHs), the lesions are limited to the skin, and the condition is benign (also known as benign neonatal haemangiomatosis). Visceral (particularly hepatic) IHs that cause life-threatening complications (also known as diffuse neonatal haemangiomatosis) appear to be rare (24). Hepatic IHs occur more commonly in infants with multiple cutaneous IHs; however, they can occur in the absence of any skin lesions. Hepatic IHs can be divided in focal, multifocal, and diffuse liver IHs. Focal and multifocal IHs are usually asymptomatic. Diffuse liver IHs may cause massive hepatomegaly with abdominal compartment syndrome, impaired ventilation secondary to splinting of the diaphragm, impaired venous return, renal vein compression, consumptive hypothyroidism, and high-output heart failure. They are associated with a high mortality rate (25, 26). Because hepatic IHs can occur with any number of cutaneous IHs, every infant requires a clinical assessment for signs of liver disease, heart failure, and/or hypothyroidism (27).

IHs can lead to permanent disfigurement (Figures 5.13a,b and 5.14a,b). Exophytic, sessile, or pedunculated IHs with a thick dermal component, particularly when in prominent locations such as

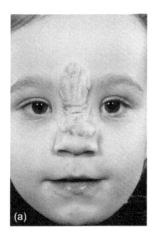 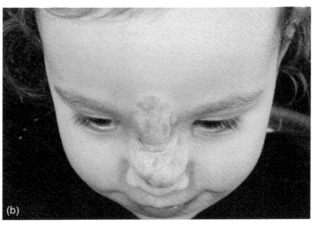

(a)    (b)

FIGURE 5.13 Stretched skin postinvolution of a mid-face IH in a 3-year-old female viewed from the front (a) and above (b).

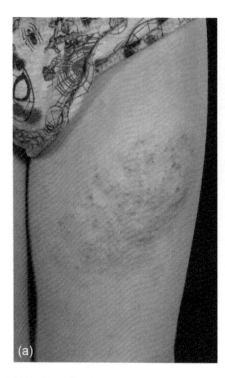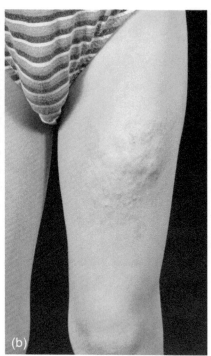

FIGURE 5.14 Residual fibrofatty tissue postinvolution of an IH of the left anterior thigh in a male child at age (a) 3 years and (b) 5 years.

the head and neck, can cause significant permanent skin change. Even after involution is complete, the prior excessive stretching of the overlying skin leads to damage in the dermal elastic tissue (anetoderma) as well as atrophy, textural change, and a persistent fibrofatty residuum (28). There is also increased recognition that parental and patient quality of life can be adversely affected by visible birthmarks and resultant scarring, particularly in areas that cannot be easily covered with clothing, such as the face, neck, arms, and hands as well as other emotionally sensitive areas, such as the breasts and genitalia (29, 30). Nasal IHs are notorious for leading to localised disfigurement and can have a profound psychological impact. They often have a deep component resting in and around the nasal cartilage. During proliferation, this leads to widening of the alar cartilage, and a round, bulbous nasal tip (28) (Figure 5.15).

## DIFFERENTIAL DIAGNOSIS

In the vast majority of infants, the diagnosis can be made on the basis of the clinical history and physical examination. At birth, IHs can be present as macular, telangiectatic patches, which is a similar appearance to a capillary malformation. Large vascular tumours that are present at birth, such as congenital haemangiomas and Kaposiform haemangioendotheliomas, are usually easily distinguishable from IHs. Vascular malformations, such as particular lymphatic and venous malformations, can sometimes mimic deep IHs. Pyogenic granulomas are commonly mistaken for IHs, but they rarely appear before the age of 4 months and, unlike IHs, frequently bleed either spontaneously or after minor trauma (Figure 5.16). It is important to distinguish an IH from a malignant tumour. Clues that are helpful in distinguishing an IH from a malignant lesion are the unique clinical history of an IH, firmness on palpation, and telangiectasias on the skin surface (31). Telangiectasias can be visible in precursor lesions and in involuted IHs; however, they are rarely present on the surface of a fully grown IH. MRI or ultrasonographic findings of high vascular flow cannot be assumed to support the diagnosis of an IH, and ultimately, a biopsy may be needed to confidently reach the diagnosis (31, 32).

## TREATMENT

The approach to treatment of an IH should be individualised, based on the size of the IH, morphology, location, potential for disfigurement, and the age of the patient. The majority of IHs do not require

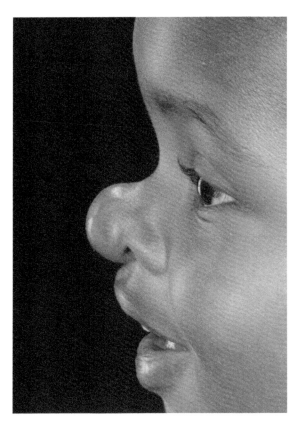

FIGURE 5.15 Residual fibrofatty tissue in an involuting nasal tip IH in a 2-year-old girl.

treatment due to their natural spontaneous involution. Indications for treatment can be divided into three main categories:

- Functional impairment
- Risk of disfigurement
- Ulceration (33)

Patients requiring treatment should be referred for treatment as early as possible, ideally before 4 weeks of age. The window of opportunity for treatment is quite narrow, as the most rapid growth occurs between 5.5 and 7.5 weeks of age (34). Treatment before the completion of the proliferative phase, which in most cases occurs by 5 months of age, may prevent poorer outcomes (24).

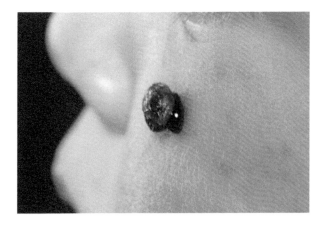

FIGURE 5.16 Pyogenic granuloma of the left cheek in a 9-month-old female.

# SYSTEMIC THERAPY

## PROPRANOLOL

In 2008, the first report of the successful use of propranolol radically changed the treatment of IHs (35). Since then, propranolol has become the first-line therapeutic agent in the management of complex IHs. The exact mechanisms of action of propranolol on IHs are still not completely understood. Recent studies indicated that a variety of mechanisms may be at play, including pericyte-mediated vasoconstriction (36), the inhibition of vasculogenesis (37), catecholamine-induced angiogenesis (38), and down-regulation of the renin–angiotensin–aldosterone axis (39).

Indications for treatment with propranolol include an IH causing or likely to cause visual obstruction, airway IH, nasal IH, lip IH, auditory canal involvement causing recurrent infection, ulcerated IH, risk of permanent disfigurement, spinal cord compression by IH, and selected liver IH (33). Absolute contraindications for treatment with propranolol include hypoglycaemic episodes, heart block, and hypersensitivity with propranolol. Relative contraindications include frequent wheezing, blood pressure, and heart rate outside the normal range for age. These patients need to be treated in conjunction with a paediatrician (33).

The prescribing physician should take a thorough history and perform a comprehensive systemic examination. An ECG is required in patients with a heart rate outside the normal range for age, a strong family history of sudden death/arrhythmia, episodes of loss of consciousness, and maternal history of connective tissue disease. A pretreatment ECHO is required in patients with a heart rate outside the normal range for age, a heart murmur detected on auscultation, and in patients with segmental IHs. Baseline glucose measurement is required if the infant is preterm, small for dates, feeding poorly, or has a history of hypoglycaemic episodes (33).

Treatment with propranolol can be initiated on an outpatient basis without monitoring of heart rate or blood pressure for infants who are older than 4 weeks with no significant comorbidities, born at term with normal birthweight, established on feeds, and demonstrating appropriate weight gain (33). Others require admission for 2–4 hours on initiation of treatment and for subsequent dose increments (<0.5 mg/kg/day). In these patients, heart rate and blood pressure are measured just before the first dose and then every 30 minutes for 2–4 hours.

The starting dose of propranolol is 1 mg/kg in three divided doses and can be increased to 2 mg/kg in three divided doses after 24 hours. The total dose can be also given in two divided doses. For preterm patients and patients with comorbidities, the dose of propranolol may need to be modified; the typical starting dose in these patients is 0.5 mg/kg in three divided doses. Individual dosing regimens for these patients are the responsibility of the local paediatrician/dermatologist (33).

Patients with segmental IHs of the head and neck and suspected PHACE syndrome should also have a cardiac assessment, including ECHO and ECG, interpreted by a paediatric cardiologist before starting propranolol. A pretreatment MRA of the head is required to exclude intracranial arterial stenosis, as propranolol can, theoretically, increase the risk of stroke if arterial stenosis is present without adequate collaterals. If it is not possible to obtain an urgent MRA, the starting dose of propranolol should be 0.5 mg/kg in three divided doses, and the dose can be increased after the MRA report has been reviewed. If arterial stenosis is shown on the MRA, the case needs to be discussed with a paediatric neurologist before increasing the dose of the propranolol.

Parents should be educated about potential adverse effects of the drug, particularly on how to prevent and recognise hypoglycaemia. Patients need to be fed regularly and propranolol needs to be stopped if there is decreased oral intake, diarrhoea, or vomiting. Propranolol should also temporarily stop if the patient has wheezing that requires treatment. Salbutamol and lidocaine (such as in teething gels) should not be used during treatment with propranolol. Sleep disturbances, or "night fright", can also occur.

During the treatment with propranolol, patients need to be assessed every 1–3 months, and there should be an appropriate dose adjustment for weight gain. The treatment with propranolol should continue beyond the proliferative phase, usually until the patient is 12–18 months of age. Rebound growth after propranolol discontinuation has been noted in 14–25% of patients (40, 41). Interestingly, rapid rebound growth within 24 hours has been noted in a patient treated with intravenous infusion of salbutamol (a beta-adrenergic receptor agonist) 10 months after stopping propranolol (42). Patients with significant rebound growth require restarting treatment with propranolol, while in milder cases, topical treatment with timolol may be sufficient.

## ATENOLOL

Atenolol is a selective beta-1-blocker and an attractive alternative to propranolol with a lower rate of sleep disturbance and broncho-reactivity, albeit with the same rate of severe adverse events as propranolol (43). In a large randomised, non-inferiority trial, 377 participants were treated with propranolol 2 mg/kg/day in three divided doses and atenolol 1 mg/kg/day in a single dose. At 6 months, a primary outcome of 'any response' was achieved in 93.7% of patients in the propranolol group and 92.5% in the atenolol group (difference, 1.2%; 95% CI, –4.1% to 6.6%) (43), suggesting atenolol may be a good alternative to propranolol, particularly in patients with sleep disturbance and wheezing.

## OTHER SYSTEMIC TREATMENTS

Historically, systemic corticosteroids were used as the primary treatment for IHs but were associated with severe adverse effects, such as gastric upset, immunosuppression, adrenal suppression, and delayed growth. They remain a treatment option if beta-blockers are contraindicated or in conjunction with beta-blockers in patients with an IH that does not respond adequately to beta-blockers. The usual starting dose is 2–3 mg/kg/day in a single dose, given in the morning. In patients treated with a high dose or prolonged course of systemic corticosteroids, a weaning plan is essential, and adrenal function tests should be discussed with an endocrinologist.

Vincristine and interferon alfa were used as an alternative to systemic steroids in patients with complex IHs in the past; however, today, they are almost never used.

# TOPICAL THERAPY

Topical beta-blockers can be beneficial in patients with small, thin, superficial IHs without a risk of functional obstruction and/or disfigurement, mainly for IHs located on the face or nappy area.

Topical beta-blockers can also be used to prevent rebound growth in patients who have stopped treatment with propranolol. Systemic absorption has been shown when timolol was used topically in the treatment of an IH. In a study of 24 children aged 2 to 35 weeks with small proliferating IHs who had topical timolol 0.5% gel applied twice a day, timolol was detected in the urine of 20 patients (44). Three patients had serum levels of timolol checked and in all three timolol was detected, although serum levels were too low to cause systemic symptoms. For that reason, treatment with topical beta-blockers in patients with large and ulcerated IHs needs to be carefully balanced against the risk of systemic absorption. In our department, we use timolol 0.5% gel-forming solution applied either as 1 drop three times a day or 2 drops twice a day, not exceeding 4 drops per day.

Topical corticosteroids are now rarely used for treatment of IHs; however, they can be useful in the treatment of ulceration. Intralesional corticosteroids are very rarely used due to the invasive nature of the therapy and attendant requirement for general anaesthetic in these young patients.

# LASER TREATMENT

In the era of oral beta-blockers, laser treatment, mainly with pulsed dye laser (PDL), is reserved for residual telangiectasias and erythema in involuted IHs. The tissue depth of the PDL penetration is 1.2 mm and, therefore, it is not aimed at decreasing the bulk of the IH. Laser treatment during the proliferation phase of the IH is associated with an increased risk of ulceration, scarring, and atrophy and is not recommended; it is not more effective than natural involution (45). Fractional laser therapy may be beneficial for residual textural skin changes after involution of the IH (46).

# SURGICAL TREATMENT

Surgery can be offered at two main points: in the early proliferative phase or late, after involution has occurred. The risk and benefits of surgical treatments should be carefully discussed with patients and parents, as the appearance of the scar may be worse than the appearance of the lesion following spontaneous involution (47). Early surgical treatment is usually reserved for removal of obstructive or ulcerated IHs if there is a contraindication to beta-blockers, such as congenital heart block. Late surgery is reserved mainly for involuted lesions with cosmetic or functional sequelae. Residual fibrofatty tissue can be removed to improve anatomical contours. Loose skin, both static and dynamic, especially any affecting facial expression, can be removed to improve both function and visual appearance. The debulking of heavy involuted IHs reduces the degree of anatomical distortion. The price of surgery is scarring and, therefore, must be performed with care and attention to the functional needs and cosmetic units of the surrounding areas. The need for and extent of surgery is likely to have been reduced by the advent of early treatment with propranolol but continues to be an important option in the multidisciplinary treatment of IH.

# TREATMENT OF ULCERATED IHs

In patients with ulcerated IHs, multimodal treatment is required, including local wound therapy, pain management, treatment of infection, prevention of bleeding, and control of proliferation. Meticulous wound care alleviates pain and prevents secondary infection and possible bleeding. Saline or gentle wound irrigating solution should be used for cleaning of the ulcer. Usually, non-adherent silicone dressing is used in combination with topical treatment such as topical antibiotics, topical corticosteroids, barrier cream, and enzyme alginogel. Oral antibiotics are sometimes needed in severe infection. Dressings are usually changed once a day, unless in the nappy area, in which case they must be changed whenever the nappy is soiled. Crusts should not be forcefully removed, as this can cause bleeding; instead, they should be treated with saline soaks a few times a day or with enzyme alginogel. For patients with ulcerated IHs who require systemic therapy, initiation of propranolol at a lower dose ($\leq 1$ mg/kg/d) should be considered, as propranolol can worsen the ulceration (48). Ulcerated IHs are usually very painful. Pain can be managed with regular paracetamol or ibuprofen, and oral morphine can be used 30–60 minutes before dressing changes.

## KEY MESSAGES

- IHs are the most common vascular tumours of childhood, affecting 4%–5% of infants. They are more common in premature or low birth-weight infants, females, and Caucasians.

- Infants with a segmental/large IH of the face, neck and/or scalp should be evaluated for PHACE syndrome.

- Segmental IHs of the gluteal cleft and lumbosacral spine extending over the midline should be investigated for underlying regional developmental abnormalities (SACRAL, LUMBAR, PELVIS).

- Ulceration is the most common IH complication, occurring in 16% of patients.

- Indications for treatment of IHs with systemic beta-blockers (propranolol or atenolol) include functional impairment, risk of disfigurement, and ulceration. The window of opportunity for treatment is quite narrow, as the most rapid growth occurs between 5.5 and 7.5 weeks of age.

- Treatment before the completion of the proliferative phase, which in most cases, occurs by 5 months of age, may prevent poorer outcomes.

- Surgical intervention in the early phase is mainly reserved for ulcerated IHs, obstructive issues of the visual axis or the airway, and later for reducing residual IH lesions.

- Laser treatment is mainly reserved for treatment of residual IH lesions.

# REFERENCES

1. Munden A, Butschek R, Tom WL, Marshall JS, Poeltler DM, Krohne SE, et al. Prospective study of infantile haemangiomas: Incidence, clinical characteristics and association with placental anomalies. *Br J Dermatol*. 2014;170(4):907–13.
2. Leaute-Labreze C, Harper JI, Hoeger PH. Infantile haemangioma. *Lancet*. 2017;390(10089):85–94.
3. Chang LC, Haggstrom AN, Drolet BA, Baselga E, Chamlin SL, Garzon MC, et al. Growth characteristics of infantile hemangiomas: Implications for management. *Pediatrics*. 2008;122(2):360–7.
4. Bauland CG, Luning TH, Smit JM, Zeebregts CJ, Spauwen PHM. Untreated hemangiomas: Growth pattern and residual lesions. *Plast Reconstr Surg*. 2011;127(4):1643–8.
5. Darrow DH, Greene AK, Mancini AJ, Nopper AJ, Section On Dermatology SOO-H, Neck S, et al. Diagnosis and management of infantile hemangioma. *Pediatrics*. 2015;136(4):e1060-104.
6. Drolet BA, Esterly NB, Frieden IJ. Hemangiomas in children. *N Engl J Med*. 1999;341(3):173–81.
7. Suh KY, Frieden IJ. Infantile hemangiomas with minimal or arrested growth: A retrospective case series. *Arch Dermatol*. 2010;146(9):971–6.
8. Endicott AA, Chamlin SL, Drolet BA, Mancini AJ, Siegel DH, Vitcov S, et al. Mapping of segmental and partial segmental infantile hemangiomas of the face and scalp. *JAMA Dermatol*. 2021;157(11):1328–34.
9. Haggstrom AN, Garzon MC, Baselga E, Chamlin SL, Frieden IJ, Holland K, et al. Risk for PHACE syndrome in infants with large facial hemangiomas. *Pediatrics*. 2010;126(2):e418–26.
10. Bayer ML, Frommelt PC, Blei F, Breur JM, Cordisco MR, Frieden IJ, et al. Congenital cardiac, aortic arch, and vascular bed anomalies in PHACE syndrome (from the International PHACE syndrome registry). *Am J Cardiol*. 2013;112(12):1948–52.
11. Hess CP, Fullerton HJ, Metry DW, Drolet BA, Siegel DH, Auguste KI, et al. Cervical and intracranial arterial anomalies in 70 patients with PHACE syndrome. *AJNR Am J Neuroradiol*. 2010;31(10):1980–6.

12. Metry DW, Haggstrom AN, Drolet BA, Baselga E, Chamlin S, Garzon M, et al. A prospective study of PHACE syndrome in infantile hemangiomas: Demographic features, clinical findings, and complications. *Am J Med Genet A*. 2006;140(9):975–86.
13. Stockman A, Boralevi F, Taieb A, Leaute-Labreze C. SACRAL syndrome: Spinal dysraphism, anogenital, cutaneous, renal and urologic anomalies, associated with an angioma of lumbosacral localization. *Dermatology*. 2007;214(1):40–5.
14. Girard C, Bigorre M, Guillot B, Bessis D. PELVIS syndrome. *Arch Dermatol*. 2006;142(7):884–8.
15. Iacobas I, Burrows PE, Frieden IJ, Liang MG, Mulliken JB, Mancini AJ, et al. LUMBAR: Association between cutaneous infantile hemangiomas of the lower body and regional congenital anomalies. *J Pediatr*. 2010;157(5):795–801 e1-7.
16. Drolet BA, Chamlin SL, Garzon MC, Adams D, Baselga E, Haggstrom AN, et al. Prospective study of spinal anomalies in children with infantile hemangiomas of the lumbosacral skin. *J Pediatr*. 2010;157(5):789–94.
17. Dadras SS, North PE, Bertoncini J, Mihm MC, Detmar M. Infantile hemangiomas are arrested in an early developmental vascular differentiation state. *Mod Pathol*. 2004;17(9):1068–79.
18. Morais CG, Alves I, Coelho J, Vilares AT, Do Bom-Sucesso M. Multifocal infantile hepatic hemangiomas complicated by consumptive hypothyroidism: The benefits of early diagnosis and treatment. *J Pediatr Hematol Oncol*. 2022; 45(2):e294–e297. doi: 10.1097/MPH.0000000000002509.
19. Darrow DH, Greene AK, Mancini AJ, Nopper AJ, Section On Dermatology SOO-H, Neck S, et al. Diagnosis and management of infantile hemangioma: Executive summary. *Pediatrics*. 2015;136(4):786–91.
20. Chamlin SL, Haggstrom AN, Drolet BA, Baselga E, Frieden IJ, Garzon MC, et al. Multicenter prospective study of ulcerated hemangiomas. *J Pediatr*. 2007;151(6):684–9, 9 e1.
21. Samuelov L, Kinori M, Rychlik K, Konanur M, Chamlin SL, Rahmani B, et al. Risk factors for ocular complications in peri-ocular infantile hemangiomas. *Pediatr Dermatol*. 2018;35(4):458–62.
22. Corbeddu M, Meucci D, Diociaiuti A, Giancristoforo S, Rotunno R, Gonfiantini MV, et al. Management of upper airway infantile hemangiomas: Experience of one Italian multidisciplinary center. *Front Pediatr*. 2021;9:717232.
23. Rahbar R, Nicollas R, Roger G, Triglia JM, Garabedian EN, McGill TJ, et al. The biology and management of subglottic hemangioma: Past, present, future. *Laryngoscope*. 2004;114(11):1880–91.
24. Metry D. Infantile hemangiomas: Epidemiology, pathogenesis, clinical features, and complications. In: *TW P*, editor. UpToDate, Waltham, MA. Accessed on July 15, 2022.
25. Christison-Lagay ER, Burrows PE, Alomari A, Dubois J, Kozakewich HP, Lane TS, et al. Hepatic hemangiomas: Subtype classification and development of a clinical practice algorithm and registry. *J Pediatr Surg*. 2007;42(1):62–7; discussion 7–8.
26. Yeh I, Bruckner AL, Sanchez R, Jeng MR, Newell BD, Frieden IJ. Diffuse infantile hepatic hemangiomas: A report of four cases successfully managed with medical therapy. *Pediatr Dermatol*. 2011;28(3):267–75.
27. Mahon C, McHugh K, Alband N, Rampling D, Sebire N, Williamson E, et al. Routine liver ultrasound screening does not alter clinical management in a cohort study of multiple cutaneous infantile haemangioma. *Br J Dermatol*. 2021;184(2):340–1.
28. Maguiness SM, Frieden IJ. Current management of infantile hemangiomas. *Semin Cutan Med Surg*. 2010;29(2):106–14.
29. Tanner JL, Dechert MP, Frieden IJ. Growing up with a facial hemangioma: Parent and child coping and adaptation. *Pediatrics*. 1998;101(3 Pt 1):446–52.
30. Fay A, Nguyen J, Waner M. Conceptual approach to the management of infantile hemangiomas. *J Pediatr*. 2010;157(6):881–8 e1-5.
31. Frieden IJ, Rogers M, Garzon MC. Conditions masquerading as infantile haemangioma: Part 2. *Australas J Dermatol*. 2009;50(3):153–68; quiz 69–70.
32. Hoornweg MJ, Theunissen CI, Hage JJ, van der Horst CM. Malignant differential diagnosis in children referred for infantile hemangioma. *Ann Plast Surg*. 2015;74(1):43–6.
33. Solman L, Glover M, Beattie PE, Buckley H, Clark S, Gach JE, et al. Oral propranolol in the treatment of proliferating infantile haemangiomas: British Society for Paediatric Dermatology consensus guidelines. *Br J Dermatol*. 2018;179(3):582–9.
34. Tollefson MM, Frieden IJ. Early growth of infantile hemangiomas: What parents' photographs tell us. *Pediatrics*. 2012;130(2):e314–20.
35. Leaute-Labreze C, Dumas de la Roque E, Hubiche T, Boralevi F, Thambo JB, Taieb A. Propranolol for severe hemangiomas of infancy. *N Engl J Med*. 2008;358(24):2649–51.
36. Lee D, Boscolo E, Durham JT, Mulliken JB, Herman IM, Bischoff J. Propranolol targets the contractility of infantile haemangioma-derived pericytes. *Br J Dermatol*. 2014;171(5):1129–37.
37. Wong A, Hardy KL, Kitajewski AM, Shawber CJ, Kitajewski JK, Wu JK. Propranolol accelerates adipogenesis in hemangioma stem cells and causes apoptosis of hemangioma endothelial cells. *Plast Reconstr Surg*. 2012;130(5):1012–21.
38. Chen XD, Ma G, Huang JL, Chen H, Jin YB, Ye XX, et al. Serum-level changes of vascular endothelial growth factor in children with infantile hemangioma after oral propranolol therapy. *Pediatr Dermatol*. 2013;30(5):549–53.
39. Itinteang T, Brasch HD, Tan ST, Day DJ. Expression of components of the renin-angiotensin system in proliferating infantile haemangioma may account for the propranolol-induced accelerated involution. *J Plast Reconstr Aesthet Surg*. 2011;64(6):759–65.
40. Wedgeworth E, Glover M, Irvine AD, Neri I, Baselga E, Clayton TH, et al. Propranolol in the treatment of infantile haemangiomas: Lessons from the European Propranolol In the Treatment of Complicated Haemangiomas (PITCH) Taskforce survey. *Br J Dermatol*. 2016;174(3):594–601.
41. Shah SD, Baselga E, McCuaig C, Pope E, Coulie J, Boon LM, et al. Rebound growth of infantile hemangiomas after propranolol therapy. *Pediatrics*. 2016;137(4):e20151754. doi: 10.1542/peds.2015-1754.
42. Knopfel N, Oesch V, Theiler M, Szello P, Weibel L. Rebound of involuted infantile hemangioma after administration of salbutamol. *Pediatrics*. 2020;145(3):e20191942. doi: 10.1542/peds.2019-1942.
43. Ji Y, Wang Q, Chen S, Xiang B, Xu Z, Li Y, et al. Oral atenolol therapy for proliferating infantile hemangioma: A prospective study. *Medicine (Baltimore)*. 2016;95(24):e3908.
44. Weibel L, Barysch MJ, Scheer HS, Konigs I, Neuhaus K, Schiestl C, et al. Topical timolol for infantile hemangiomas: Evidence for efficacy and degree of systemic absorption. *Pediatr Dermatol*. 2016;33(2):184–90.
45. Batta K, Goodyear HM, Moss C, Williams HC, Hiller L, Waters R. Randomised controlled study of early pulsed dye laser treatment of uncomplicated childhood haemangiomas: Results of a 1-year analysis. *Lancet*. 2002;360(9332):521–7.
46. Brightman LA, Brauer JA, Terushkin V, Hunzeker C, Reddy KK, Weiss ET, et al. Ablative fractional resurfacing for involuted hemangioma residuum. *Arch Dermatol*. 2012;148(11):1294–8.
47. McHeik JN, Renauld V, Duport G, Vergnes P, Levard G. Surgical treatment of haemangioma in infants. *Br J Plast Surg*. 2005;58(8):1067–72.
48. Fernandez Faith E, Shah S, Witman PM, Harfmann K, Bradley F, Blei F, et al. Clinical features, prognostic factors, and treatment interventions for ulceration in patients with infantile hemangioma. *JAMA Dermatol*. 2021;157(5):566–72.

# Other Vascular Tumours

# 6

Claire O'Neill and Lea Solman

## INTRODUCTION

Vascular tumours result from the proliferation of endothelial and other vascular cells. The proliferative ability of vascular tumours ranges from benign local growth with potential local disfigurement to locally aggressive tumours with tissue destruction, and, in rare cases, malignancies with the potential for distant metastases. Vascular tumours can also induce systemic life-threatening complications such as Kasabach–Merritt phenomenon or heart failure.

Aside from infantile haemangiomas, most vascular tumours are rare entities and can be challenging to diagnose and treat, as there are no standardised evidence-based management guidelines.

## CONGENITAL HAEMANGIOMAS

Congenital haemangiomas (CHs) are rare benign vascular lesions present at birth. They have been reported to occur in 0.3% of newborns (1). They are distinct from the much more common infantile haemangiomas (IHs) in their clinical presentation, behaviour, and histologic features. Three subtypes have been described according to their natural spontaneous involution and likely represent a spectrum of the same condition, although, clinically, they behave very differently: rapidly involuting congenital haemangiomas (RICHs), partially involuting congenital haemangiomas (PICH), and non-involuting congenital haemangiomas (NICHs). Some teams have argued that CHs may represent slow proliferative malformations based on their genetic basis. Somatic activating mutations in *GNAQ* and *GNA11* have been identified in a subset of CHs (2).

### CLINICAL PRESENTATION AND DIAGNOSIS

CHs occur fully formed at birth and are sometimes diagnosed *in utero* as a vascular mass on antenatal ultrasound scans. They are localised and contained to one area, most commonly the head, neck, and limbs, but can be found anywhere on the body (Figure 6.1). Solid organ involvement is rare, although RICHs have a predilection for the liver. Multifocal and segmental lesions have been reported (3, 4).

In most cases, the diagnosis is based on the clinical history and examination. NICHs are typically relatively sessile lesions with a benign appearance. They present as a violaceous cutaneous mass, often with a peripheral pale rim and coarse overlying telangiectasia. In contrast, RICHs can be extremely large and are often initially mistaken for an aggressive soft tissue tumour. They are usually exophytic and can be deep red or purple in colour. The overlying skin is often thinned and taut and ulceration can occur. Large cutaneous and visceral CHs can be associated with life-threatening high-output cardiac failure due to the high volume of flow through these markedly vascular lesions. RICHs of the liver are often occult in the first few days of life and only diagnosed when the child is examined for the cause of their cardiac compromise. Liver RICHs tend to be

DOI: 10.1201/9781003257417-6

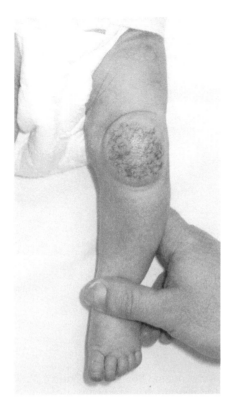

FIGURE 6.1 Congenital haemangioma of the left knee in a 2-week-old girl.

exceedingly large and can cause respiratory compromise due to splinting of the diaphragm and even abdominal compartment syndrome (5).

At first presentation, the child's full blood count, clotting profile, and D-dimer level should be checked due to the risk of associated transient thrombocytopenia and coagulopathy and should be repeated if clinically warranted.

Imaging may be required when the diagnosis is unclear. CHs are typically confined to the skin and subcutaneous fat. On ultrasound, they are less homogeneous than IHs and demonstrate marked vascularity with numerous vessels, high velocity blood flow, venous lakes, and, rarely, calcifications (6, 7) (Figure 6.2). On magnetic resonance imaging (MRI), they demonstrate hyperintensity on T2-weighted

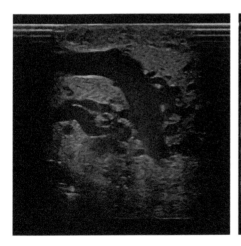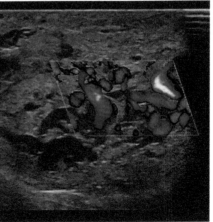

FIGURE 6.2 Ultrasound images of a RICH in a 1-day-old male, showing a heterogeneous soft tissue mass with large central vessels, venous lakes, and marked vascular flow.

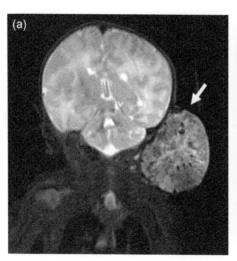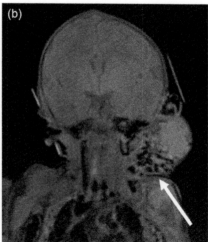

FIGURE 6.3 MRI of a 6-day-old child with a RICH in the left side of the neck. (a) Coronal T2-weighted fat-suppressed image showing the heterogenous mass (short arrow). The central black dots represent blood vessels. (b) Coronal T1-weighted fat-suppressed image demonstrating the poorly defined deep margin of the lesion and the very large feeding vessels and draining veins at its base in the neck (long arrow).

sequences, heterogeneous enhancement, and flow voids (Figure 6.3). They are usually distinguishable from IHs by their less well-defined margins, heterogeneous stroma, and ectatic irregular vascular channel, often looking more like an aggressive tumour than an IH on imaging (7).

If the diagnosis is uncertain or a malignant tumour is suspected, biopsy should be considered. A core needle biopsy sample is usually sufficient. Biopsies should be performed in a controlled environment by an experienced interventional radiology or surgical team because of the risk of bleeding, and haematology advice should always be sought prior to the procedure to ensure the child's coagulation profile is normalised as much as possible during the procedure.

All types of CH show similar histological features in their early stages with histological findings diverging later, as the lesions either persist or regress. CHs exhibit nodules or lobules of capillary-size vessels lined by bland endothelial cells, usually dermal or subcutaneous, and initially similar in appearance to IHs. As RICHs regress or involute, the lesions may demonstrate central loss of the capillary lobules with a relative increase in fibrous tissue, with or without haemosiderin pigment. Residual, obsolete draining veins can persist. Characteristically, the endothelial cells of CHs do not express GLUT1, although patchy podoplanin may be expressed in some lesions in infants (8). The fact that CHs are GLUT-1 negative allows immediate histological differentiation from IHs if the diagnosis is unclear.

## NATURAL HISTORY

The behaviour pattern of CHs over time varies by subtype. RICHs undergo spontaneous involution (Figures 6.4 and 6.5). Involution of large RICHs almost invariably results in a residual patch of telangiectatic vessels, atrophy, or absence of subcutaneous fat and often a leash of obsolete draining veins. PICHs partially involute over time and then stabilise in size and appear somewhat similar to their initial presentation but flattened (Figure 6.6). This process of spontaneous involution generally occurs in the first year of life. In contrast, NICHs do not undergo any involution and will grow in proportion with the child (Figure 6.7). They may have some progressive features in late childhood, with further growth and pain in adolescence, for example (Figure 6.8) (9). The diagnosis of RICH over PICH or NICH is usually made with time.

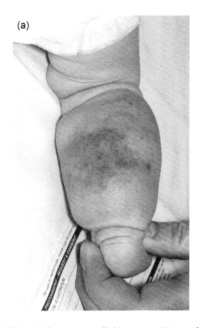
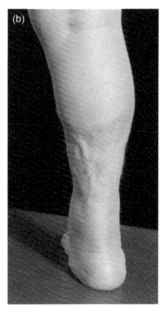

FIGURE 6.4 Rapidly involuting congenital haemangioma of the right calf, at age (a) 8 weeks and (b) 3 years.

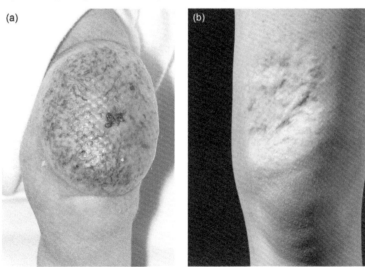

FIGURE 6.5 Rapidly involuting congenital haemangioma of the left anterior thigh, at age (a) 2 weeks and (b) 16 years.

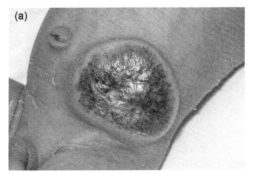
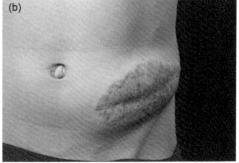

FIGURE 6.6 Partially involuting congenital haemangioma of the left lower abdomen in a male child at age (a) birth and (b) 4 years post-partial surgical resection.

Congenital Haemangiomas

51

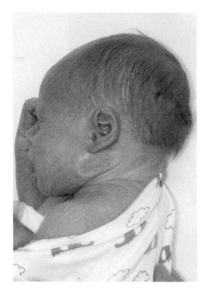

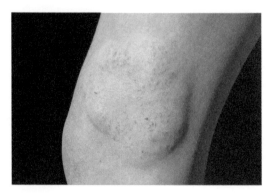

FIGURE 6.8 Non-involuting congenital haemangioma of the left lateral thigh in a 10-year-old female.

FIGURE 6.7 Non-involuting congenital haemangioma of the left lateral jaw in a 1-week-old male infant.

## COMPLICATIONS

Due to their high-flow nature, RICHs can be associated with life-threatening complications. The presence of ulceration, crusting, or erosions in a CH is an ominous sign that can precede episodes of severe or even life-threatening bleeding (Figure 6.9) (10). These patients require close follow-up and meticulous wound care with non-adherent dressings, barrier cream, and topical antibiotics.

Localised consumptive coagulopathy and thrombocytopenia is common in large RICHs, although less severe than the true Kasabach–Merritt phenomenon observed with Kaposiform haemangioendothelioma. It usually resolves in the first few weeks of life (11, 12). Large CHs can lead to functional impairment or the risk for permanent disfigurement, depending on their location. Pain is a frequent feature of NICHs, postulated to be secondary to local vasoconstriction (13). In addition, persisting large draining vessels in the skin surrounding a CH may with time become ectatic and symptomatic (Figure 6.10).

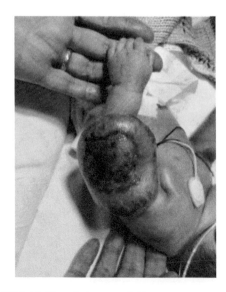

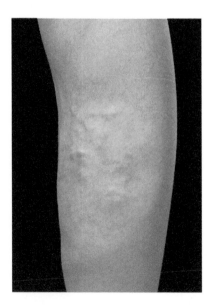

FIGURE 6.9 Ulcerated congenital haemangioma of the left upper arm in a 4-day-old male infant.

FIGURE 6.10 Residual prominent draining veins in a congenital haemangioma of the right calf in a 14-year-old female.

## MANAGEMENT

Management of CHs is dictated by their size, location, natural history, and the presence of complications. For most children, simple observation is indicated, with parental education given around the risk of ulceration, especially for large CHs.

Infants with large RICHs may require neonatal intensive care and interventional measures such as embolisation. Coagulopathy may be treated with fibrinogen replacement therapy (fresh frozen plasma, cryoprecipitate, and fibrinogen concentrate). Platelet transfusion should be used judiciously, only to treat haemorrhage or to cover patients undergoing a surgical procedure, because of the underlying consumptive process which may be exacerbated with platelet transfusions (14). High-output cardiac failure is usually managed sufficiently with supportive measures such as diuretics and respiratory support, but in rare cases, partial embolisation of the tumour may be required. This intervention aims to decrease the volume of blood through the lesion and reduce the right heart strain, simply as a temporising measure until the natural involution of the RICH occurs (6). Embolisation is a technically challenging procedure in a critically unwell, fluid-overloaded neonate and should be undertaken with extreme caution; liquid embolics or coils should be used and particles avoided at all costs. An alternative approach to devascularise superficial lesions is to temporarily compress the lesion, in effect squeezing the large blood volume out of the abnormal vascular bed so that the child's haemodynamics can stabilise. This must be done with utmost caution and reviewed daily, as it carries the risk of inadvertent skin necrosis which can cause critical haemorrhage. But it may play a role in cases where embolisation carries too high a risk. Surgical excision should be seen as an option of last resort and can almost always be avoided.

Ulceration in CHs can result in life-threatening bleeding; thus, it is important any signs of skin breakdown are assessed by a specialist team with experience in wound care and in optimising tissue viability in patients with vascular anomalies.

Currently, there are no medical therapies proven to improve the clinical course of CHs. There is no evidence that beta-blockers accelerate involution of CHs.

At a later stage, atrophic or redundant tissue after involution of a RICH may benefit from surgical intervention for functional or aesthetic reasons. A persistent PICH and NICH which may be causing disfigurement and pain may also benefit from surgery (Figure 6.11).

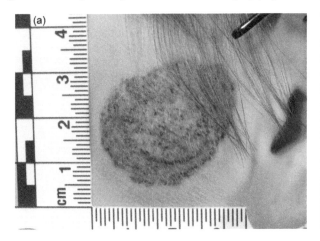 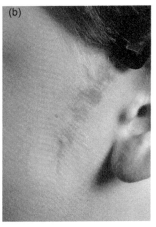

FIGURE 6.11  Congenital haemangioma of the left cheek of an 8-year-old male, (a) pre-excision and (b) post-excision.

# PYOGENIC GRANULOMAS

Pyogenic granulomas (or lobular capillary haemangiomas) are relatively common, acquired benign vascular tumours of the skin and mucosa (15, 16). They usually appear as a solitary, red, pedunculated papule that is very friable and bleeds easily with small trauma (Figures 6.12 and 6.13). The size rarely exceeds one centimetre. Mature lesions are polypoid or pedunculated and have a "collarette" of scale at the base of the lesion, which may help to make the diagnosis (17). The size rarely exceeds one centimetre. They are usually located in the craniofacial region or extremities. They are typically superficial, but deeper lesions occur and can be challenging to diagnose (18). History and physical examination are usually sufficient for diagnosis.

Pyogenic granulomas are also frequently reported to develop on a background of other vascular anomalies such as capillary malformations or arteriovenous malformations, with second somatic hits in RAS-MAPK pathway genes identified in lesional tissue (Figure 6.14) (19). They may be associated with medication use such as retinoids (20).

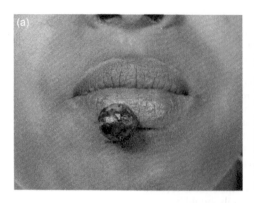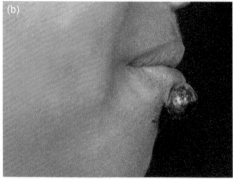

FIGURE 6.12 Classic pyogenic granuloma of the right lower lip in an 11-year-old male (a) front view and (b) side view.

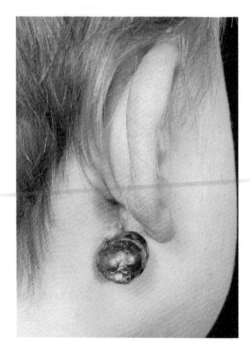

FIGURE 6.13 Large post-auricular pyogenic granuloma in an 8-year-old male.

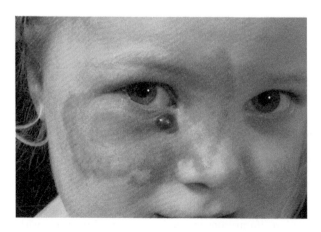

FIGURE 6.14 Pyogenic granuloma arising from a left facial capillary malformation in a 2-year-old girl.

Histologically, pyogenic granulomas demonstrate some similar features to capillary haemangiomas, such as lobules of capillary-size vascular channels with plump endothelial cells, separated by loose or fibrotic stroma. However, pyogenic granulomas usually affect superficial areas and have a characteristic low-power architecture, showing lateral "collarettes" of epithelium. In addition, variable degrees of inflammation are usually co-existent, and there may even be ulceration with superficial granulation tissue formation. GLUT1 immunostaining is negative. Somatic activating mutations in *NRAS/KRAS/BRAF* genes have been found in some pyogenic granulomas (21, 22).

## TREATMENT

Some pyogenic granulomas may regress spontaneously; however, most lesions require surgery due to their propensity to bleed. Complete excision is often required, as recurrence can occur if less invasive techniques are used, such as shave removal, curettage, or laser photocoagulation (23, 24). Topical beta-blockers have been used with some success to treat pyogenic granulomas; however, evidence is limited to case reports and small cases series (25).

# OTHER HAEMANGIOMAS

## EPITHELIOID AND SPINDLE CELL HAEMANGIOMAS

These are rare, benign vascular tumours which can occur in childhood. They are usually small and well circumscribed. There are no widely agreed management guidelines, and surgical resection is the first-line treatment option, when possible.

Epithelioid haemangiomas are most often found in the skin and soft tissues but are also frequently reported in liver and bone, where they have lytic properties. They present as painful swellings and can be multifocal. They may occur following trauma. Surgical resection can be curative. Sirolimus has been used as a medical treatment (26, 27).

Spindle cell haemangiomas present as painful, red or brown deep cutaneous or subcutaneous nodules, mostly found on the extremities. They have also been reported to affect other tissues, viscera, and bone (28, 29). They can be multifocal. On histopathology, cavernous blood spaces are surrounded by areas of spindle cell proliferation (30). Spindle cell haemangiomas can also be observed in Maffuci syndrome, associated with benign enchondromas and a predisposition to malignancy (31). Treatment is surgical resection, but they have a tendency to recur.

# LOCALLY AGGRESSIVE VASCULAR TUMOURS

## KAPOSIFORM HAEMANGIOENDOTHELIOMA AND TUFTED ANGIOMA

Kaposiform haemangioendotheliomas (KHEs) and tufted angiomas (TAs) are considered to be part of the same disease spectrum, as they have overlapping clinical and histological features. They are rare vascular tumours classified as locally aggressive or borderline and usually present in infancy and early childhood. They can be associated with life-threatening complications such as Kasabach–Merritt phenomenon (KMP), which is characterised by consumptive coagulopathy with thrombocytopenia and hypofibrinogenemia, leading to a high risk of intravascular coagulation and bleeding. KHEs and TAs can be challenging to treat haematologically (see Chapter 3). A consensus document for the treatment of KMP with steroids and vincristine was produced in 2013 but, today, is challenged by the growing recent evidence of successful outcomes with the use of sirolimus as a first-line treatment.

### Clinical Presentation and Diagnosis

The precise incidence of these lesions has not been evaluated, but KHE and TA are considered to be rare. Both KHEs and TAs present as localised, firm, indurated vascular masses, occurring from birth or presenting later in infancy and early childhood (Figures 6.15–6.17). Some cases have been reported to present in adulthood (32). They are typically highly vascularised, violaceous, indurated plaques which can progressively swell or, in some cases, present as expansive masses at birth. Hypertrichosis and hyperhidrosis can also be present. Their margins are relatively well-defined, depending on the tissue level affected.

In general, TAs are considered superficial lesions compared to KHEs, which are usually more invasive. KHEs and TAs can involve any part of the body, although some studies have demonstrated a predilection for neck, axilla, groin, and extremities. Approximately 10% of KHE do not involve skin. The

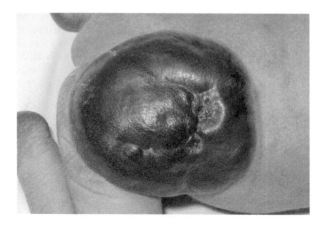

FIGURE 6.15 Kaposiform haemangioendothelioma of the right lower back and buttock in a 3-day-old male.

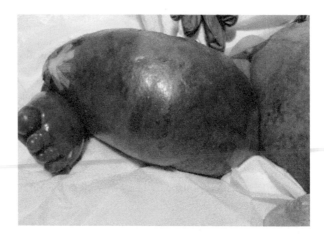

FIGURE 6.16 Kaposiform haemangioendothelioma of the left lower leg in a 3-day-old female with Kasabach–Merritt phenomenon.

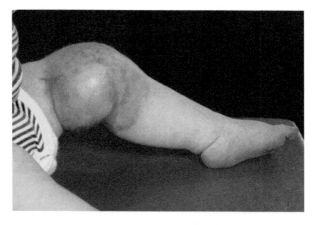

FIGURE 6.17 Tufted angioma of the left knee and upper thigh in a 10-month-old female.

most common extracutaneous location is in the retroperitoneum, followed by muscle and bone, which, understandably, leads to a delay in diagnosis (33–35). There have been reports of multifocal lesions (36, 37) but no reports of distant metastasis.

Both KHE and TA can episodically present with engorgement with an associated violaceous colour change and swelling and pain secondary to known trigger factors such as trauma or concomitant systemic infections (38, 39). KHE may also exhibit dramatic swelling and colour change in the context of KMP onset.

Imaging has value both in identifying that the imaging features are not those of a haemangioma and in delineating the extent of the lesion. Ultrasound of a KHE or TA reveals markedly heterogeneous parenchyma with swathes of very dense, echogenic tissue interspersed between more hypoechoic disease. The parenchyma can cast a significant acoustic shadow, and calcification is possible. The lesions have internal vascularity but not generally on the scale of that seen in CHs or proliferative IHs (Figure 6.18). MRI usually reveals a plaque of homogeneous T2-bright lesion infiltrating the subcutaneous soft tissues, which enhances relatively uniformly (Figure 6.19). The lesion often crosses tissue planes and can invade bone. The striking imaging feature of these lesions is the associated subcutaneous oedema, which either overlies the lesion or exists at its margins (40, 41) (Figure 6.4).

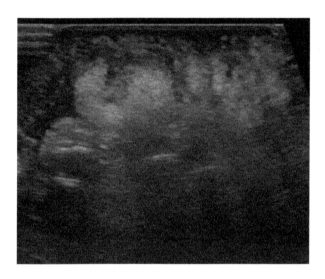

FIGURE 6.18 Ultrasound image of a KHE in a 10-month-old child, showing echogenic deposits deep to more hypoechoic tissue. Note the acoustic shadow deep to the echogenic parenchyma.

In cases of diagnostic uncertainty, a biopsy is recommended. The risk of bleeding in the setting of KMP is often perceived as a barrier to early biopsy; support from a haematologist is key. Histological confirmation is crucial in atypical or particularly aggressive lesions to exclude critical differential diagnoses such as infantile sarcomas. The biopsy should be performed by an experienced team with the coordination of surgeons or interventional radiologists and haematologists. It is important to ensure that any sample is taken from the dense central parenchyma; sampling of the peripheral oedematous soft tissues is often non-diagnostic.

The histological features of KHEs and TAs have significant overlap, and both are considered to be of the same neoplastic spectrum (42). They have, historically, been differentiated clinically, with less severe superficial involvement ascribed to TAs and multiple levels of infiltration ascribed for KHEs. TAs are characterised by the presence of scattered tufts and rounded lobules of closely packed capillaries in "cannonball" distribution (Figure 6.20a). They demonstrate histological features of a non-encapsulated vascular lesion composed of cellular lobules, usually in the dermis and subcutaneous tissue, which, on low-power examination, may have rounded outlines. The cellular component is composed of capillary type vessels with plump but bland endothelial cells. Typically, at the periphery of the lobules, a slit-like intravascular space is seen as well as a generic expression of endothelial markers CD31/34, lesional cells of TA as GLUT1 negative. D2-40 immunostaining demonstrates focal expression of vascular endothelium, usually at the periphery of the lobules (Figure 6.20b).

KHE represents a closely related lesion, which also exhibits similar histological features, including vascular lobules but with more prominent spindle cells, prominent flattened vascular spaces, diffuse

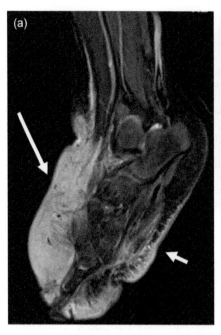
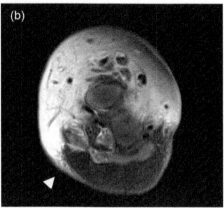

FIGURE 6.19 MRI of a KHE infiltrating the foot of a 16-month-old child. (a) Sagittal T2-weighted fat-suppressed image showing a thick rind of echogenic tissue encasing the foot (long arrow). Note the subcutaneous oedema in the sole (short arrow). (b) Axial T2-weighted fat-suppressed image illustrating how the lesion infiltrates the muscle planes. The margins are indistinct (arrowhead).

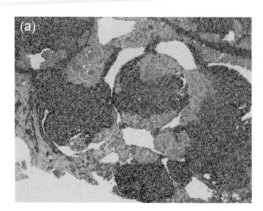
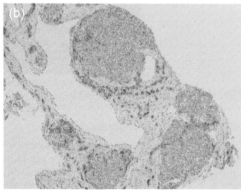

FIGURE 6.20 Photomicrographs of a TA: (a) H&E staining, original magnification x100, and (b) D2-40 staining, original magnification x100, demonstrating a characteristic low-power appearance of multiple cellular nodules surrounded by abnormal vascular spaces into which the nodules extend. The cellular areas show spindle cells and slit-like vascular spaces similar to KHEs. However, with TAs, D2-40 immunostaining typically highlights the peripheral endothelium only.

infiltration pattern, and widespread, uniform expression of D2-40 (Figure 6.21a,b). Thrombi or platelet aggregates within the lobular capillaries are often identified along with scattered hemosiderin pigment. The presence of lymphangiomatosis and sheet-like patterns of growth and spindle cells similar to those in Kaposi sarcoma have, historically, been features differentiating KHEs from TAs; however, this is thought to be a spectrum. KHE is negative for HHV-8 expression, differentiating it from Kaposi sarcoma, which it can resemble morphologically.

KHE and TA have identical immunophenotyping to both vascular (CD31, CD34, and VEGFR-3) and lymphatic (D2-40, LYVE1, and PROX1) endothelium markers with progressive angiogenesis and lymphangiogenesis (43). They are negative for GLUT-1.

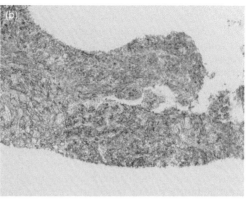

FIGURE 6.21 Photomicrographs of a case of KHE: (a) H&E staining, original magnification x100, and (b) D2-40 staining, original magnification x100, demonstrating a non-encapsulated lesion composed of lobules of cellular spindle cells, which on higher power, demonstrate numerous slit-like vascular channels but with no atypia; characteristically, there is diffuse expression of D2-40 in the majority of the lesional endothelial cells.

## Kasabach–Merritt Phenomenon

Up to 70% of patients with KHE and 10% of patients with TA develop KMP (44). KMP is a life-threatening coagulopathy characterised by profoundly low platelets ($< 25 \times 10^9/L$), low fibrinogen, and low levels of red blood cells. The low red blood cells are due to a microangiopathic haemolytic anaemia. Laboratory evaluation should include a full blood count, coagulation panel, and D-dimer level. Coagulation studies will reveal a prolonged prothrombin time (PT) and partial thromboplastin time (PTT), hypofibrinogenaemia, and raised D-dimer levels.

KMP is often marked by rapid enlargement of the tumour itself as platelet aggregation occurs (Figure 6.22). The mortality rate associated with KMP is estimated to be 10%–30% (45). KMP seems to occur more frequently in association with larger KHEs and those located in the retroperitoneum, intrathoracic region, or with extensive involvement of more than one region (46, 47). In these cases, proactive treatment of KHE is highly recommended to mitigate the risk of KMP (48).

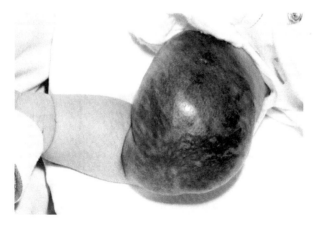

FIGURE 6.22 Kaposiform haemangioendothelioma of the left upper leg in a 3-day-old male with Kasabach–Merritt phenomenon.

Though the precise mechanism underlying KMP has not yet been established, it has been theorised that the convoluted angioarchitecture within the tumour promotes platelet and protein trapping, leading to platelet activation and fibrinogen consumption (49). This theory has been supported by positive staining of entrapped platelets within the lumen and consumption of radio-labelled fibrinogen (33). KMP is discussed in further detail in Chapter 3.

## Other Complications

The morbidity of KHEs and TAs can extend beyond the initial complications associated with KMP. Due to the locally aggressive nature of the tumour with infiltration of muscle, joints, and bones as well as fibrotic tissue remodelling, patients often suffer painful musculoskeletal complications and functional impairment.

## Treatment

Close monitoring without intervention may be an option for small, localised lesions without KMP and which do not impair the child's function (50). Treatment of symptomatic or growing KHEs and TAs should be initiated as soon as possible but becomes urgent in the context of KMP. While thrombocytopenia may be profound, life-threatening haemorrhage is rare. Platelet transfusion is usually not recommended except in cases of active bleeding or before/during surgical procedures (33). Platelet transfusion may potentiate platelet trapping and lead to further platelet activation and tumour growth. Symptomatic anaemia should be treated with red blood cell transfusion. Fresh frozen plasma, cryoprecipitate, or fibrinogen concentrate may be administered to correct fibrinogen levels.

Treatment of the underlying KHE is critical in the management of KMP. In rare cases, surgical resection may be considered as a definitive treatment for KHEs if this is anatomically possible. Unfortunately, the extensive and infiltrative nature of most of these tumours, together with the associated coagulopathy, renders this option impossible. Embolisation may be of value for partial correction of the coagulopathy if target dominant feeding vessels are accessible. Embolisation acts to exclude some of the abnormal endothelial bed likely to be inducing KMP (51) or, in some instances, to manage high-output heart failure associated with large KHEs. Early use of surgery or embolisation can be considered as rescue therapies while waiting for medical therapies to take effect or in refractory life-threatening situations.

Medical management guidelines of KMP in KHE were introduced in 2013 and recommend the use of vincristine and steroids as the first-line treatment (52), but more recent evidence suggests sirolimus, an inhibitor of mTOR, is also an effective first-line therapy. One meta-analysis in 2016 suggested vincristine led to a better response rate than any other treatment modality, but further studies have confirmed good response rates from sirolimus (53–55). Although sirolimus and vincristine have never been compared prospectively, some retrospective studies have now more recently reported higher response rates with sirolimus (56, 57). Therefore, teams around the world, including our centre, now use sirolimus as a first-line treatment in the majority of patients with symptomatic KHE or TA.

Combined therapies with either short courses of steroids and/or vincristine in the initial period of onset of KMP are also still indicated and could offer even higher response rates (58).

Sirolimus has the benefit of ease of administration and relatively good tolerance and safety profile. However, it is important to note that sirolimus has immunomodulating properties, and cases of severe infection, such as meningitis leading to brain damage and infant deaths, have been reported on treatment, thus, stressing the need for close monitoring of sirolimus therapy and education of patients and their families (59).

Sirolimus is often prescribed at a dose of 0.8 mg/m$^2$ twice a day with target whole blood trough levels of 5–15 ng/mL. This standardised dosage for use in paediatric vascular anomalies was widely adopted after results of a study on the use of sirolimus in children with vascular anomalies (52). Low range levels of sirolimus may be sufficient to control KMP (60), but better results with regard to tumour shrinkage may be obtained with a level between 10–15 (61). For KMP responsive to sirolimus, time to response is, on average, 1–2 weeks, and by 4 weeks, platelets and haemoglobin have usually normalised (35, 37).

For KHEs and TAs without KMP, as mentioned above, active close monitoring without intervention can be an option. However, if the lesion is expanding or causes functional impairment or pain, intervention is often necessary. Long-term treatment with sirolimus seems to be effective to address these complications. The duration of treatment should be individualised to the patient's response. Sirolimus target serum levels will be based on therapeutic objectives and patient tolerance.

Superficial lesions, in most cases identified as TA, have been treated with topical mTOR inhibitors to control symptoms with good outcomes (62).

## Natural History

Following initial treatment and stabilisation of life-threatening or debilitating complications, KHEs and TAs will continue to evolve and fluctuate in colour, size, and texture, with transient episodes of growth and exacerbations. Monitoring for these changes will be important, as it may portend the onset of KMP and guide further treatment plans. Specific triggers have been reported to stimulate KHE and TA activity, such as infection, vaccinations, trauma, surgery, growth spurts, puberty, and hormonal changes. Examples of KHE reactivation in adolescence have been reported (Figure 6.23) (63).

KHEs and TAs may spontaneously decrease in size without medical intervention (Figure 6.24) or following intensive treatment (Figure 6.25).

From the literature, it seems that there is no complete and permanent resolution of these lesions, and a residual form of KHE and TA will remain in a quiescent state (64). They then appear as flat vascular markings resembling capillary malformations or as a focal area of telangiectasia, mild swelling, and fibrosis.

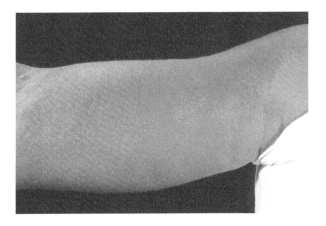

FIGURE 6.23 Acute flare of a right arm Kaposiform haemangioendothelioma in a 13-year-old female.

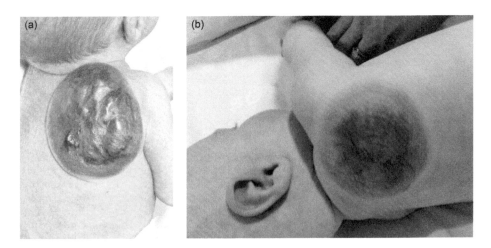

FIGURE 6.24 Spontaneous involution of a Kaposiform haemangioendothelioma of the right upper back in a male infant shown at (a) 11 days of age and (b) 3 months of age.

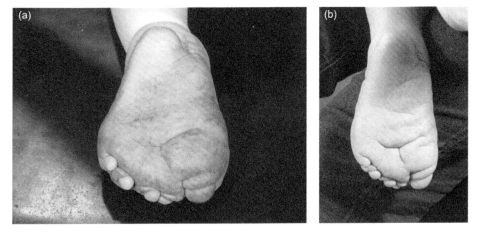

FIGURE 6.25 Kaposiform haemangioendothelioma of the left foot in a female infant treated with sirolimus and vincristine shown at age (a) 16 months and (b) 33 months.

**TABLE 6.1**  Other haemangioendotheliomas

| Entity | Pathology | Clinical Presentation |
|---|---|---|
| Retiform haemangioendothelioma | Dermis subcutis<br>Vessels lines by protruding endothelial cells, net-like vascular composition<br>Endothelial markers positive | Young adults, occasionally children<br>Limb and trunk |
| Papillary intralymphatic angioendothelioma | Dermis subcutis<br>Intravascular growth of hobnail endothelial cells that form intraluminal papillary projections | Also known as Dabska tumour<br>Raised firm slow-growing purplish skin nodules or plaques<br>Some lesions associated with vascular malformations |
| Pseudomyogenic (or sarcoma-like) haemangioendothelioma | Loose fascicules of epithelioid and spindle cells<br>Abundant eosinophil cytoplasm<br>Positive for endothelial markers | Young men<br>Soft tissue mass/nodule<br>Can be multifocal<br>Dermis, subcutis, and bone |
| Composite haemangioendothelioma | Combined benign and malignant vascular components (epithelioid, retiform, and spindle cell) | All age groups<br>Extremities |

Residual KHEs and TAs involving joints, bones, and muscle may impair function with muscle contractures or bony deformities. Residual KHEs and TAs may cause chronic or intermittent pain. Sirolimus is now increasingly used for the long-term treatment of KHEs and TAs with chronic pain and function impairment (65). Pain relief in patients treated with sirolimus may, in part, be explained by the reduction in vascularisation (66).

Lymphoedema may occur downstream of the lesion, particularly in large lesions involving an extremity (67).

Early involvement of physiotherapists may help to support the management of contractures and pain. Compression garments may be beneficial for lymphoedema.

## OTHER HAEMANGIOENDOTHELIOMAS

Several other haemangioendothelioma-type tumours have been described to occur only very rarely in children. Their features are sometimes borderline with those of angiosarcomas, and their histopathological diagnosis can be challenging. They have a potential to be locally aggressive and can have locoregional extension with local lymph node involvement but seldom metastasise, although there have been some such reports for each subtype.

The diagnosis is made histologically with endothelial cell abnormalities and endothelial or lymphatic cell markers. Histological analysis needs to identify atypia or high index mitosis to rule out malignant tissue.

First-line treatment is surgical resection, when possible, but they have a tendency to recur locally. Radiation therapy can be an option for localised tumours which are not amenable for surgery. Sirolimus and other chemotherapies have been used for aggressive or metastatic disease.

## MALIGNANT VASCULAR TUMOURS

Malignant vascular tumours are exceptionally rare in childhood. Children with a clinical diagnosis and histological diagnosis of vascular tumour atypia and malignancy should be referred to and managed by a paediatric oncology team. Management will follow paediatric soft tissue sarcoma guidelines, which may involve surgery, chemotherapy, and radiation therapy. For this chapter to be comprehensive, epithelioid haemangioendothelioma and angiosarcoma are briefly discussed.

## EPITHELIOID HAEMANGIOENDOTHELIOMA

Epithelioid haemangioendothelioma (EHE) is a vascular tumour of the sarcoma family, usually found in the liver, lung, bone, and soft tissue. These can be indolent tumours or have an aggressive course and present with metastases. Their peak incidence is in middle-age adults. Histologically, the lesions are characterised by clusters of arterioles filled with damaged endothelial cells (epithelial-like), surrounded by inflammatory cells that are primarily composed of eosinophils. These lesions lack mitotic activity and are reactive rather than neoplastic. They can be divided into two subtypes: cellular epithelioid haemangioma and atypical epithelioid haemangioma. The first exhibits more than 50% sheet-like growth of tumour cells. Atypical epithelioid haemangioma, on the other hand, displays more nuclear pleomorphism, solid growth, focal necrosis, and infiltrative growth and often has FOSB fusions. Angiolymphoid hyperplasia with eosinophilia subtype of epithelioid haemangioma may be non-neoplastic due to a lack of the FOS or FOSB gene rearrangement. Immunohistochemically, the tumour cells are positive for FOSB in approximately 50% of epithelioid haemangioma (including angiolymphoid hyperplasia with eosinophilia subtype).

Gene fusion anomalies have been identified in several studies (pathognomonic WWTR1 and CAMTA1 fusion). One multicentre study reported the outcome of 24 patients between the ages of 2 and 26 years with EHE; in the majority, there was multiorgan disease and a progressive course was seen in two-thirds of cases.

mTOR inhibitors have recently been reported for the treatment of EHE with some results of progression-free outcomes. More aggressive disease is treated as per angiosarcoma guidelines (68, 69).

## ANGIOSARCOMAS

Angiosarcomas are very rare malignant vascular tumours that can arise at any site but most commonly in soft tissue. They represent less than 1% of soft tissue sarcomas. They most commonly present in older adults, typically on the face and neck, but cases have been described in children. Long-standing lymphedema is a known risk factor for developing angiosarcomas, which may be the most relevant point in vascular anomalies patient populations, but other risk factors have been reported, such as radiation exposure or vinyl chloride exposure. The prognosis of angiosarcomas is poor, with studies reporting overall survival rates of 25%–30% at 5 years (70, 71).

There are case reports of hepatic IHs undergoing malignant transformation to angiosarcomas. Recent guidelines advise imaging follow-up of hepatic IHs to monitor for evidence of involution. If their involution is atypical, or if any hepatic symptoms arise, it is important to consider this rare but severe outcome (72, 73).

## A NOTE ON SOFT TISSUE LESIONS WITH INCREASED VASCULARITY

Malignant tumours of any tissue will often display increased or atypical vascularity and may, initially, be interpreted as a vascular anomaly, but vascularity alone should not dissuade the clinical team from considering the possibility of malignancy.

---

## KEY MESSAGES

- Any atypical and/or acquired and/or progressive vascular lesion that does not have the typical features or clinical history of an IH or CH should be biopsied.

- Pyogenic granulomas also have pathognomonic clinical features in most cases and will most likely go through an excision-diagnosis pathway.

- If a KHE or TA is suspected, the patient should be screened for thrombocytopenia and clotting abnormalities.

- Vascular malignant tumours are rare and have a poor prognosis.

# REFERENCES

1. Kanada KN, Merin MR, Munden A, Friedlander SF. A prospective study of cutaneous findings in newborns in the United States: Correlation with race, ethnicity, and gestational status using updated classification and nomenclature. *J Pediatr.* 2012 Aug;161(2):240–5.
2. Ayturk UM, Couto JA, Hann S, Mulliken JB, Williams KL, Huang AY, et al. Somatic activating mutations in GNAQ and GNA11 are associated with congenital hemangioma. *Am J Hum Genet.* 2016 Apr 7;98(4):789–95.
3. Mulliken JB, Bischoff J, Kozakewich HPW. Multifocal rapidly involuting congenital hemangioma: A link to chorangioma. *Am J Med Genet A.* 2007 Dec 15;143A(24):3038–46.
4. Smith RJ, Metry D, Deardorff MA, Heller E, Grand KL, Iacobas I, et al. Segmental congenital hemangiomas: Three cases of a rare entity. *Pediatr Dermatol.* 2020 May;37(3):548–53.
5. Roebuck D, Sebire N, Lehmann E, et al. Rapidly involuting congenital haemangioma (RICH) of the liver. *Pediatr Radiol.* 2012 42:308–314.
6. Waelti SL, Rypens F, Damphousse A, Powell J, Soulez G, Messerli M, et al. Ultrasound findings in rapidly involuting congenital hemangioma (RICH) – Beware of venous ectasia and venous lakes. *Pediatr Radiol.* 2018 Apr;48(4):586–93.
7. Gorincour G, Kokta V, Rypens F, Garel L, Powell J, Dubois J. Imaging characteristics of two subtypes of congenital hemangiomas: Rapidly involuting congenital hemangiomas and non-involuting congenital hemangiomas. *Pediatr Radiol.* 2005 Dec;35(12):1178–85.
8. North PE, Waner M, James CA, Mizeracki A, Frieden IJ, Mihm MC. Congenital nonprogressive hemangioma: A distinct clinicopathologic entity unlike infantile hemangioma. *Arch Dermatol.* 2001 Dec;137(12):1607–20.
9. Hua C, Wang L, Jin Y, Chen H, Ma G, Gong X, et al. A case series of tardive expansion congenital hemangioma: A variation of noninvoluting congenital hemangioma or a new hemangiomatous entity? *J Am Acad Dermatol.* 2021 May;84(5):1371–7.
10. Powell J, Blouin MM, David M, Dubois J. Bleeding in congenital hemangiomas: Crusting as a clinical predictive sign and usefulness of tranexamic acid. *Pediatr Dermatol.* 2012;29(2):182–5.
11. Weitz NA, Lauren CT, Starc TJ, Kandel JJ, Bateman DA, Morel KD, et al. Congenital cutaneous hemangioma causing cardiac failure: A case report and review of the literature. *Pediatr Dermatol.* 2013;30(6):e180–190.
12. Liang MG, Frieden IJ. Infantile and congenital hemangiomas. *Semin Pediatr Surg.* 2014 Aug;23(4):162–7.
13. Lee PW, Frieden IJ, Streicher JL, McCalmont T, Haggstrom AN. Characteristics of noninvoluting congenital hemangioma: A retrospective review. *J Am Acad Dermatol.* 2014 May;70(5):899–903.
14. Al Malki A, Al Bluwi S, Malloizel-Delaunay J, Mazereeuw-Hautier J. Massive hemorrhage: A rare complication of rapidly involuting congenital hemangioma. *Pediatr Dermatol.* 2018 May;35(3):e159–60.
15. Patrice SJ, Wiss K, Mulliken JB. Pyogenic granuloma (lobular capillary hemangioma): A clinicopathologic study of 178 cases. *Pediatr Dermatol.* 1991 Dec;8(4):267–76.
16. Pagliai KA, Cohen BA. Pyogenic granuloma in children. *Pediatr Dermatol.* 2004;21(1):10–3.
17. Sarwal P, Lapumnuaypol K. Pyogenic Granuloma. In: StatPearls [Internet]. Treasure Island (FL): StatPearls Publishing; 2022 [cited 2022 Nov 25]. Available from: http://www.ncbi.nlm.nih.gov/books/NBK556077/
18. Putra J, Rymeski B, Merrow AC, Dasgupta R, Gupta A. Four cases of pediatric deep-seated/subcutaneous pyogenic granuloma: Review of literature and differential diagnosis. *J Cutan Pathol.* 2017 Jun;44(6):516–22.
19. Baselga E, Wassef M, Lopez S, Hoffman W, Cordisco M, Frieden IJ. Agminated, eruptive pyogenic granuloma-like lesions developing over congenital vascular stains. *Pediatr Dermatol.* 2012;29(2):186–90.
20. Benedetto C, Crasto D, Ettefagh L, Nami N. Development of periungual pyogenic granuloma with associated paronychia following isotretinoin therapy: A case report and a review of the literature. *J Clin Aesthetic Dermatol.* 2019 Apr;12(4):32–6.
21. Lim YH, Douglas SR, Ko CJ, Antaya RJ, McNiff JM, Zhou J, et al. Somatic activating RAS mutations cause vascular tumors including pyogenic granuloma. *J Invest Dermatol.* 2015 Jun;135(6). Available from: https://pubmed.ncbi.nlm.nih.gov/25695684/
22. Groesser L, Peterhof E, Evert M, Landthaler M, Berneburg M, Hafner C. BRAF and RAS mutations in sporadic and secondary pyogenic granuloma. *J Invest Dermatol.* 2016 Feb;136(2):481–6.
23. Lee J, Sinno H, Tahiri Y, Gilardino MS. Treatment options for cutaneous pyogenic granulomas: A review. *J Plast Reconstr Aesthetic Surg JPRAS.* 2011 Sep;64(9):1216–20.
24. Patrizi A, Gurioli C, Dika E. Pyogenic granulomas in childhood: New treatment modalities. *Dermatol Ther.* 2015;28(5):332.
25. Neri I, Baraldi C, Balestri R, Piraccini BM, Patrizi A. Topical 1% propranolol ointment with occlusion in treatment of pyogenic granulomas: An open-label study in 22 children. *Pediatr Dermatol.* 2018 Jan;35(1):117–20.
26. Liu KX, Duggan EM, Al-Ibraheemi A, Shaikh R, Adams DM. Characterization of long-term outcomes for pediatric patients with epithelioid hemangioma. *Pediatr Blood Cancer.* 2019 Jan;66(1):e27451.
27. Liu KX, Duggan EM, Al-Ibraheemi A, Shaikh R, Adams DM. Characterization of long-term outcomes for pediatric patients with epithelioid hemangioma. *Pediatr Blood Cancer.* 2019 Jan;66(1):e27451.
28. Nimkar A, Mandel M, Buyuk A, Stavropoulos C, Naaraayan A. Spindle cell hemangioma of the lung: A case report. *Cureus.* 2022 Jan;14(1):e21191.
29. Huang C, Zhang H, Guan L, Luo J. Rare spindle cell hemangioma of bone: Case report and literature review. *Radiol Case Rep.* 2022 Mar;17(3):886–90.
30. Enjolras O, Mulliken JB, Kozakewich HPW. Vascular Tumors and Tumor-Like Lesions. In: Mulliken JB, Burrows PE, Fishman SJ, editors. *Mulliken and Young's Vascular Anomalies: Hemangiomas and Malformations* [Internet]. Oxford University Press; 2013 [cited 2022 Nov 25]. Available from: https://doi.org/10.1093/med/9780195145052.003.0008
31. Prokopchuk O, Andres S, Becker K, Holzapfel K, Hartmann D, Friess H. Maffucci syndrome and neoplasms: A case report and review of the literature. *BMC Res Notes.* 2016 Feb 27;9:126.

32. Mentzel T, Mazzoleni G, Dei Tos AP, Fletcher CD. Kaposiform hemangioendothelioma in adults. Clinicopathologic and immunohistochemical analysis of three cases. *Am J Clin Pathol*. 1997 Oct;108(4):450–5.

33. Mahajan P, Margolin J, Iacobas I. Kasabach-Merritt phenomenon: Classic presentation and management options. *Clin Med Insights Blood Disord*. 2017;10:1179545X17699849.

34. Kuo C, Warren M, Malvar J, Miller JM, Shah R, Navid F, et al. Kaposiform hemangioendothelioma of the bone in children and adolescents. *Pediatr Blood Cancer*. 2022 Jan;69(1):e29392.

35. Ji Y, Chen S, Li L, Yang K, Xia C, Li L, et al. Kaposiform hemangioendothelioma without cutaneous involvement. *J Cancer Res Clin Oncol*. 2018 Dec;144(12):2475–84.

36. Wang Z, Yao W, Sun H, Dong K, Ma Y, Chen L, et al. Sirolimus therapy for kaposiform hemangioendothelioma with long-term follow-up. *J Dermatol*. 2019 Nov;46(11):956–61.

37. Cohen OG, Florez-Pollack S, Finn LS, Larijani M, Jen M, Treat J, et al. Multifocal kaposiform hemangioendothelioma in a newborn with confirmatory histopathology. *Pediatrics*. 2022 Nov 1;150(5):e2022056293.

38. Peng S, Yang K, Xu Z, Chen S, Ji Y. Vincristine and sirolimus in the treatment of kaposiform haemangioendothelioma. *J Paediatr Child Health*. 2019 Sep;55(9):1119–24.

39. Ji Y, Chen S, Yang K, Xia C, Peng S. Development of Kasabach-Merritt phenomenon following vaccination: More than a coincidence? *J Dermatol*. 2018 Oct;45(10):1203–6.

40. Hu PA, Zhou ZR. Clinical and imaging features of kaposiform hemangioendothelioma. *Br J Radiol*. 2018 Jun;91(1086):20170798.

41. Ryu YJ, Choi YH, Cheon JE, Kim WS, Kim IO, Park JE, et al. Imaging findings of kaposiform hemangioendothelioma in children. *Eur J Radiol*. 2017 Jan;86:198–205.

42. Le Huu AR, Jokinen CH, Rubin BP, Mihm MC, Weiss SW, North PE, et al. Expression of prox1, lymphatic endothelial nuclear transcription factor, in kaposiform hemangioendothelioma and tufted angioma. *Am J Surg Pathol*. 2010 Nov;34(11):1563–73.

43. Ji Y, Chen S, Yang K, Xia C, Li L. Kaposiform hemangioendothelioma: Current knowledge and future perspectives. *Orphanet J Rare Dis*. 2020 Feb 3;15(1):39.

44. Putra J, Gupta A. Kaposiform haemangioendothelioma: A review with emphasis on histological differential diagnosis. *Pathology (Phila)*. 2017 Jun;49(4):356–62.

45. Oza VS, Mamlouk MD, Hess CP, Mathes EF, Frieden IJ. Role of sirolimus in advanced kaposiform hemangioendothelioma. *Pediatr Dermatol*. 2016;33(2):e88–92.

46. Croteau SE, Liang MG, Kozakewich HP, Alomari AI, Fishman SJ, Mulliken JB, et al. Kaposiform hemangioendothelioma: Atypical features and risks of Kasabach-Merritt phenomenon in 107 referrals. *J Pediatr*. 2013 Jan;162(1):142–7.

47. Sarkar M, Mulliken JB, Kozakewich HP, Robertson RL, Burrows PE. Thrombocytopenic coagulopathy (Kasabach-Merritt phenomenon) is associated with kaposiform hemangioendothelioma and not with common infantile hemangioma. *Plast Reconstr Surg*. 1997 Nov;100(6):1377–86.

48. Schmid I, Klenk AK, Sparber-Sauer M, Koscielniak E, Maxwell R, Häberle B. Kaposiform hemangioendothelioma in children: A benign vascular tumor with multiple treatment options. *World J Pediatr WJP*. 2018 Aug;14(4):322–9.

49. O'Rafferty C, O'Regan GM, Irvine AD, Smith OP. Recent advances in the pathobiology and management of Kasabach-Merritt phenomenon. *Br J Haematol*. 2015 Oct;171(1):38–51.

50. Osio A, Fraitag S, Hadj-Rabia S, Bodemer C, de Prost Y, Hamel-Teillac D. Clinical spectrum of tufted angiomas in childhood: A report of 13 cases and a review of the literature. *Arch Dermatol*. 2010 Jul;146(7):758–63.

51. Brill R, Uller W, Huf V, Müller-Wille R, Schmid I, Pohl A, et al. Additive value of transarterial embolization to systemic sirolimus treatment in kaposiform hemangioendothelioma. *Int J Cancer*. 2021 May 1;148(9):2345–51.

52. Drolet BA, Trenor CC, Brandão LR, Chiu YE, Chun RH, Dasgupta R, et al. Consensus-derived practice standards plan for complicated kaposiform hemangioendothelioma. *J Pediatr*. 2013 Jul;163(1):285–91.

53. Adams DM, Trenor CC, Hammill AM, Vinks AA, Patel MN, Chaudry G, et al. Efficacy and safety of sirolimus in the treatment of complicated vascular anomalies. *Pediatrics*. 2016 Feb;137(2):e20153257.

54. Wang Z, Li K, Dong K, Xiao X, Zheng S. Successful treatment of Kasabach-Merritt phenomenon arising from kaposiform hemangioendothelioma by sirolimus. *J Pediatr Hematol Oncol*. 2015 Jan;37(1):72–3.

55. Kai L, Wang Z, Yao W, Dong K, Xiao X. Sirolimus, a promising treatment for refractory kaposiform hemangioendothelioma. *J Cancer Res Clin Oncol*. 2014 Mar;140(3):471–6.

56. Boccara O, Puzenat E, Proust S, Leblanc T, Lasne D, Hadj-Rabia S, et al. The effects of sirolimus on Kasabach-Merritt phenomenon coagulopathy. *Br J Dermatol*. 2018 Feb;178(2):e114–6.

57. Peng S, Yang K, Xu Z, Chen S, Ji Y. Vincristine and sirolimus in the treatment of kaposiform haemangioendothelioma. *J Paediatr Child Health*. 2019 Sep;55(9):1119–24.

58. Ji Y, Chen S, Zhou J, Yang K, Zhang X, Xiang B, et al. Sirolimus plus prednisolone vs sirolimus monotherapy for kaposiform hemangioendothelioma: A randomized clinical trial. *Blood*. 2022 Mar 17;139(11):1619–30.

59. Ying H, Qiao C, Yang X, Lin X. A case report of 2 Sirolimus-related deaths among infants with kaposiform hemangioendotheliomas. *Pediatrics*. 2018 Apr;141(Suppl 5):S425–9.

60. Harbers VEM, van der Salm N, Pegge SAH, van der Vleuten CJM, Verhoeven BH, Vrancken SLAG, et al. Effective low-dose sirolimus regimen for kaposiform haemangioendothelioma with Kasabach-Merritt phenomenon in young infants. *Br J Clin Pharmacol*. 2022 Jun;88(6):2769–81.

61. Shan Y, Tian R, Gao H, Zhang L, Li J, Xie C, et al. Sirolimus for the treatment of kaposiform hemangioendothelioma: In a trough level-dependent way. *J Dermatol*. 2021 Aug;48(8):1201–9.

62. Burleigh A, Kanigsberg N, Lam JM. Topical rapamycin (sirolimus) for the treatment of uncomplicated tufted angiomas in two children and review of the literature. *Pediatr Dermatol*. 2018 Sep;35(5):e286–90.

63. Schaefer BA, Wang D, Merrow AC, Dickie BH, Adams DM. Long-term outcome for kaposiform hemangioendothelioma: A report of two cases. *Pediatr Blood Cancer*. 2017 Feb;64(2):284–6.

64. Enjolras O, Mulliken JB, Wassef M, Frieden IJ, Rieu PN, Burrows PE. et al. Residual lesions after Kasabach-Merritt phenomenon in 41 patients. *J Am Acad Dermatol*. 2000 Feb;42(2 Pt 1):225–35.

65. Oza VS, Mamlouk MD, Hess CP, Mathes EF, Frieden IJ. Role of sirolimus in advanced kaposiform hemangioendothelioma. *Pediatr Dermatol*. 2016;33(2):e88–92.

66. Iacobas I, Simon ML, Amir T, Gribbin CE, McPartland TG, Kaufman MR. et al. Decreased vascularization of retroperitoneal kaposiform hemangioendothelioma induced by treatment with sirolimus explains relief of symptoms. *Clin Imaging*. 2015;39(3):529–32.

67. Ji Y, Chen S, Xia C, Zhou J, Jiang X, Xu X, et al. Chronic lymphedema in patients with kaposiform hemangioendothelioma: Incidence, clinical features, risk factors and management. *Orphanet J Rare Dis*. 2020 Nov 7;15(1):313.

68. Rosenberg A, Agulnik M. Epithelioid hemangioendothelioma: Update on diagnosis and treatment. *Curr Treat Options Oncol*. 2018 Mar 15;19(4):19.

69. Cournoyer E, Al-Ibraheemi A, Engel E, Chaudry G, Stapleton S, Adams DM. Clinical characterization and long-term outcomes in pediatric epithelioid hemangioendothelioma. *Pediatr Blood Cancer.* 2020 Feb;67(2):e28045.
70. Ferrari A, Casanova M, Bisogno G, Cecchetto G, Meazza C, Gandola L, et al. Malignant vascular tumors in children and adolescents: A report from the Italian and German Soft Tissue Sarcoma Cooperative Group. *Med Pediatr Oncol.* 2002 Aug;39(2):109–14.
71. Deyrup AT, Miettinen M, North PE, Khoury JD, Tighiouart M, Spunt SL, et al. Pediatric cutaneous angiosarcomas: A clinicopathologic study of 10 cases. *Am J Surg Pathol.* 2011 Jan;35(1):70–5.
72. Grassia KL, Peterman CM, Iacobas I, Margolin JF, Bien E, Padhye B, et al. Clinical case series of pediatric hepatic angiosarcoma. *Pediatr Blood Cancer.* 2017 Nov;64(11). doi: 10.1002/pbc.26627.
73. Jeng MR, Fuh B, Blatt J, Gupta A, Merrow AC, Hammill A, et al. Malignant transformation of infantile hemangioma to angiosarcoma: Response to chemotherapy with bevacizumab. *Pediatr Blood Cancer.* 2014 Nov;61(11):2115–7.

Other Vascular Tumours

# 7 Capillary Malformations

Claire O'Neill and Mary Glover

## INTRODUCTION

Capillary malformations (CM) are estimated to affect about 0.3%–0.5% of newborns, occurring equally in males and females (1). They present as flat pink to violaceous marks, which may be well demarcated, diffuse, reticulate, focal, or multifocal and either isolated or associated with other anomalies (Figures 7.1–7.3). Historically, understanding has been hampered by confusing terminology but has been greatly aided by the demonstration that many of these vascular lesions and related anomalies arise from activating somatic mutations in the PI3K/AKT/mTOR or RAS-MAPK pathways.

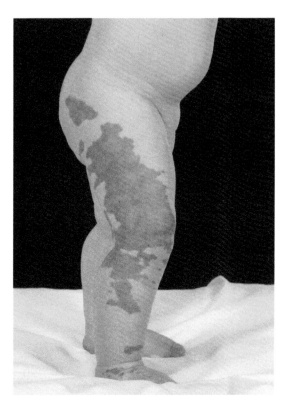

FIGURE 7.1 Geographic capillary malformation of the left lateral lower thigh and anterior knee in a 10-month-old female.

DOI: 10.1201/9781003257417-7

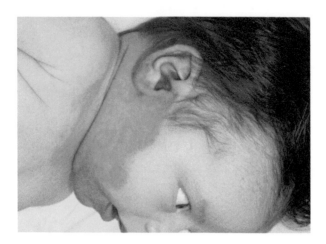

FIGURE 7.2 Capillary malformation of the left lower face, neck, and upper chest in a newborn.

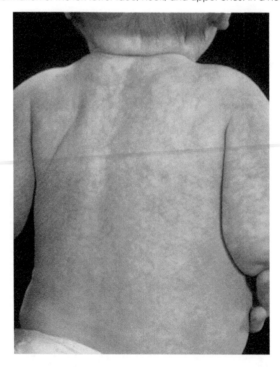

FIGURE 7.3 Extensive reticulate capillary malformation shown here on the back and bilateral arms in an 11-month-old female.

Biopsies of such lesions are rarely performed but demonstrate scattered dilated capillary-type vessels in the superficial dermis. With increasing age, CM demonstrates more prominent, abnormally distributed, ectatic vessels with capillary and venular morphology in the superficial and deep dermis.

## CLASSIFICATION

Several important classification schemes have been proposed (2, 3). In this chapter, we have drawn on these to describe six patterns of CMs: nevus simplex (NS), port-wine stain (PWS), reticulate CM, geographic CM, CM–arteriovenous malformation (CM-AVM), and cutis marmorata telangiectatica congenita (CMTC).

# NAEVUS SIMPLEX

Naevus simplex (NS), also known as stork mark, angel's kiss, or salmon patch, is a common, benign CM of newborns thought to arise from a delay in cellular maturation. The name is misleading, as it is not a true naevus.

It presents as flat pink to red patches with irregular borders, most commonly presenting as a symmetrical patch on the glabella often in a 'V' shape and on the nape of the neck (Figure 7.4). The marks are frequently more visible when straining or with changes in temperature and emotion. Those on the face usually fade in infancy, but those on the nape of the neck tend to persist. Some children present with more extensive patches which may include the nose, philtrum, scalp, and midline of the back. This more extensive pattern is sometimes termed NS complex (4).

Differentiation of NS from PWS may be difficult, particularly in the newborn. NS tends to be less well demarcated and centrally located, whilst PWS have clear margins and are more likely to be located away from the midline.

Typical NS does not require any investigation, but infants with lumbosacral NS associated with a lipoma, aplasia cutis, pits, or localised hypertrichosis require spinal imaging to exclude spinal dysraphism (5).

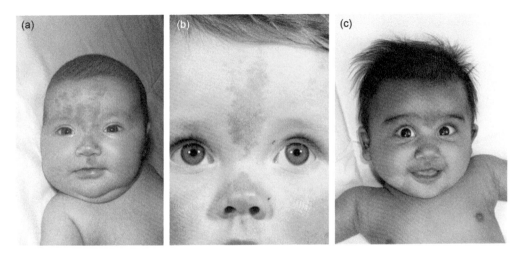

FIGURE 7.4 (a) Naevus simplex of the forehead, glabella, nose, and philtrum in an 8-week-old female. (b) Naevus simplex of the glabella and nasal tip in an 8-month-old female. (c) Naevus simplex of the glabella and philtrum in a 3-month-old female.

# PORT-WINE STAIN

Port-wine stains (PWS) are generally well demarcated, solid pink, red, or purple marks, frequently unilateral and segmental, that can occur anywhere on the body (Figure 7.5). Facial PWS, in particular, may darken and thicken overtime secondary to continuing vascular ectasia (6) and, in some cases, may be associated with overgrowth of soft tissue and bone (Figure 7.6) (7).

Eczematous dermatitis of the overlying skin, probably arising from disruption of the skin barrier by vascular stasis and/or excessive production of proinflammatory makers by the ectatic capillary vessels, is relatively common and usually responds well to topical steroids (8).

Pyogenic granulomas may arise, particularly from the cheek area of a PWS. It is thought that laser treatment may act as a trigger in some cases (9).

Most isolated PWS lesions are the result of somatic *GNAQ* or *GNA11* mutations (10).

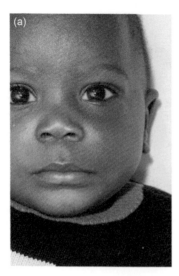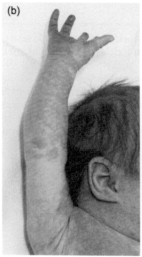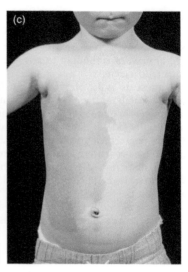

FIGURE 7.5 (a) Left facial port-wine stain in a 7-month-old male. (b) Port-wine stain of the right upper chest, arm, and hand in a 3-week-old female. (c) Segmental port-wine stain of the right anterolateral trunk in a 2-year-old male.

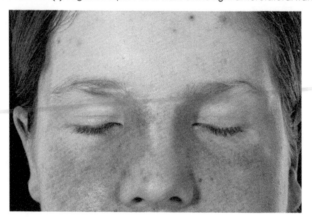

FIGURE 7.6 Thickened port-wine stain of the face post-laser therapy in a 15-year-old girl.

## STURGE–WEBER SYNDROME

PWS of the forehead region may be associated with leptomeningeal angiomatosis and ocular vascular malformations leading to buphthalmos and glaucoma (11), referred to as Sturge–Weber syndrome (SWS) (Figure 7.7).

Historically, it was thought that CMs distributed in the V1 (ophthalmic) branch of the trigeminal nerve territory presented an increased risk of the presence of SWS. It is now clear that the risk is not related to trigeminal nerve territory but is, instead, determined by involvement of the tissues arising from the embryological frontal placode, with PWS involving the forehead area from the midline to a line joining the outer canthus of the eye to the top of the ear (12).

Glaucoma is the most frequent ocular manifestation of SWS, usually developing in early childhood and resulting from vascular malformations of the anterior chamber. Choroidal haemangiomas also occur in about 50% of SWS patients. Both manifestations can lead to visual loss (13).

Leptomeningeal malformations are usually ipsilateral and involve the parietal and occipital lobes. The main clinical manifestations are seizures, slowly progressive hemiparesis, headaches, transient ischemic episodes, developmental delay, and behavioural issues (11).

Up to a third of patients have a clinical diagnosis of autism, with a larger proportion showing social communication difficulties (14).

Brain magnetic resonance imaging (MRI) with contrast is the imaging modality of choice. Findings include leptomeningeal enhancement, choroid plexus enlargement, venous anomalies, extensive deep venous vessels, and cortical atrophy (Figure 7.8). These changes are more evident after one year of age (15).

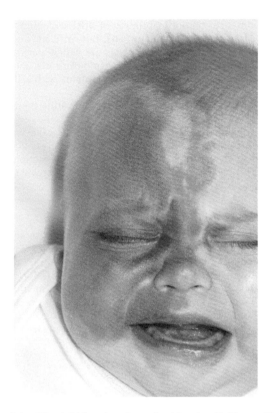

FIGURE 7.7 Facial port-wine stain of the right face in a 4-month-old male with Sturge–Weber syndrome.

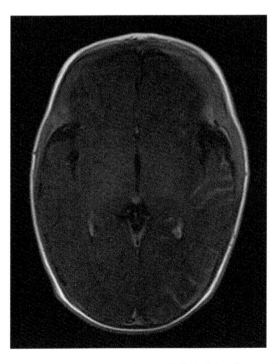

FIGURE 7.8 Image from an axial T1-weighted contrast enhanced MR study in a 7-year-old child, showing increased enhancement of the leptomeninges overlying the left hemisphere in keeping with a pial angioma.

There is, currently, no consensus on optimal timing of MRI screening. Routine screening was not recommended by U.S. 2021 consensus statement (16), but, instead, early referral to a neurologist was recommended for at-risk patients. However, MRIs are widely performed in the first month to year of life for those at risk of SWS to aid diagnosis, inform prognosis, and enable early intervention. We recommend routine screening with brain MRI for all infants with a PWS in the forehead region (12, 17).

The genetic basis of SWS has been identified as somatic activating mutations in the genes *GNAQ*, *GNA11*, and *GNB2* (18, 19).

Infants at risk of glaucoma should be referred for ophthalmological assessment, with review every 3 months in the first year of life and annually thereafter (20).

Management may include pre-symptomatic neuroprotective interventions such as prophylactic anti-epileptic drug treatment (21). Low-dose prophylactic aspirin may decrease the frequency of cerebrovascular events (22).

## PHAKOMATOSIS PIGMENTOVASCULARIS (PPV)

Phakomatosis pigmentovascularis (PPV) is characterised by the co-existence of a vascular lesion, commonly a CM, and a pigmentary lesion (Figure 7.9). PPV may be associated with extracutaneous features, including glaucoma, choroidal haemangioma, uveal melanoma, seizures, and development delay. PPV has been associated with activating somatic mutations in *GNA11*, *GNAQ*, and *PTPN11* (23).

Treatment of PWS is usually with pulsed dye laser (Figure 7.10). Small lesions can be treated using local anaesthetic cream to reduce discomfort but larger areas, and skin close to the eye, will usually require general anaesthesia. Multiple treatments are required to produce a satisfactory result, and recurrence is common. Infants with Fitzpatrick skin phototype 1-2 typically have the best response, and facial PWS respond better than those on the distal limbs.

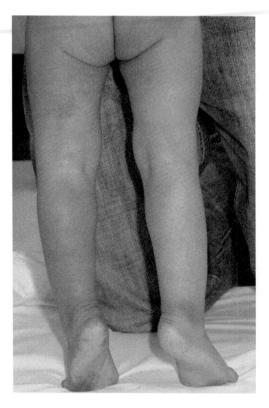

FIGURE 7.9 Phacomatosis pigmentovascularis cesioflammea type: overlapping areas of dermal melanocytosis and capillary malformation in the buttocks and lower legs of a 1-year-old boy.

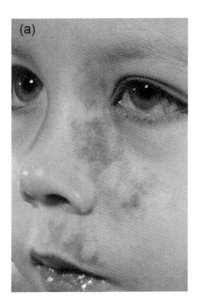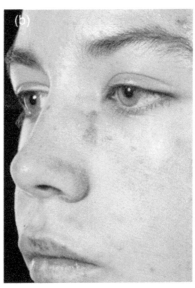

FIGURE 7.10 Left facial port-wine stain (a) pre-laser therapy at 2 years of age and (b) post-laser therapy at 14 years of age in a male child/adolescent.

# RETICULATE CAPILLARY MALFORMATION

These tend to be poorly defined, pink or red 'lace-like' networks that are often widespread (Figures 7.3 and 7.11). They may be isolated or associated with undergrowth or overgrowth, as in diffuse CM with overgrowth (DCMO) or with macrocephaly/megalencephaly.

In DCMO, the overgrowth is proportional and non-progressive and not always co-located with the CM. DCMO is caused by somatic activating mutations in *PIK3CA* mutations (24) and forms part of the *PIK3CA*-related overgrowth spectrum, which is discussed in more detail in Chapter 12.

Megalencephaly-CM syndrome (MCAP) refers to the co-occurrence of diffuse reticulate and/or blotchy CMs, characteristically including the philtrum, with macrocephaly (Figure 7.12). There is often also asymmetric overgrowth, syndactyly, and polydactyly. Development delay and learning difficulties may co-exist (25).

Neuroimaging findings include megalencephaly, thickening of the corpus callosum, Chiari malformation, ventriculomegaly/hydrocephaly, cerebral asymmetry, and polymicrogyria (26).

MCAP mainly arises from somatic *PIK3CA*-related overgrowth spectrum (PROS) (27).

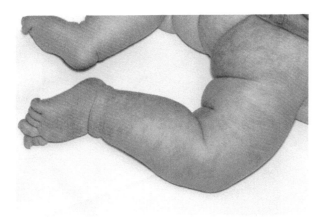

FIGURE 7.11 Reticulate capillary malformation of the lower legs in a 4-month-old female.

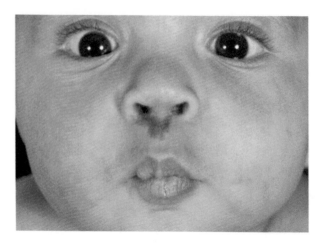

FIGURE 7.12 Capillary malformation of the upper philtrum in a 7-month-old male with megalencephaly-capillary malformation syndrome.

# CAPILLARY MALFORMATIONS WITH GEOGRAPHIC BORDERS

Geographic CMs are characterised by well demarcated, angular margins. They tend to be dark red to purple and are not widespread, generally involving only part of a body zone (Figures 7.1 and 7.13). They are associated with lymphatic malformations, which are usually evident as haemorrhagic vesicles and papules, and with venous malformations and overgrowth. Somatic activating mutations in *PIK3CA* can be found in most cases.

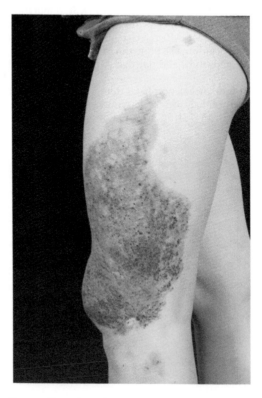

FIGURE 7.13 Geographic capillary malformation of the left lateral knee and thigh in a 5-year-old female.

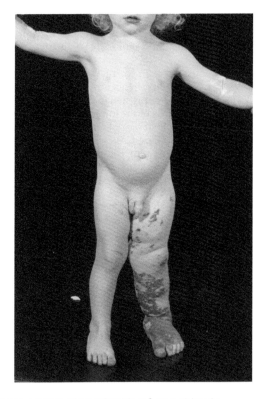

FIGURE 7.14 Klippel–Trenaunay syndrome of the left leg in a 2-year-old male.

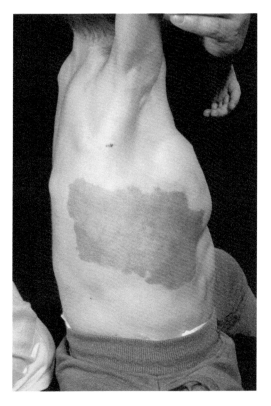

FIGURE 7.15 Capillary malformation of the right lateral chest wall in CLOVES syndrome in a 3-year-old male.

Geographic CMs are most frequently encountered as part of Klippel–Trenaunay syndrome (KTS), which refers to the triad of CM with geographic borders, venous malformation, and overgrowth of a limb, with or without a lymphatic malformation (Figure 7.14). Somatic activating mutations in *PIK3CA* can be found in most cases.

CLOVES syndrome (congenital lipomatous overgrowth, vascular malformations including CMs, epidermal naevus and scoliosis/spinal/skeletal anomalies) frequently includes geographic type CMs, often overlying lipomatous areas (Figure 7.15). Somatic activating mutations in *PIK3CA* can be found in most cases.

CLAPO syndrome features geographic CMs of the lower lip and chin region, with lymphatic malformation of the head and neck and asymmetry and partial or generalised overgrowth (28).

Management of patients with geographic type CMs will depend on the location of the lesion, any associated anomalies, and the child's presenting symptoms. Orthopaedic input is required for leg length discrepancy, tailored imaging and interventional radiology for management of venous and lymphatic anomalies, and plastic surgery for debulking and reconstruction.

There has been considerable debate concerning the need for screening for Wilms' tumour for infants and children with *PIK3CA*-related overgrowth. The most recent recommendations from the American Association for Cancer Research are that screening is not required because cancer risk estimates are below 1% (29).

# CAPILLARY MALFORMATION–ARTERIOVENOUS MALFORMATION (CM-AVM)

Capillary malformation–arteriovenous malformation (CM-AVM) is an autosomal dominant condition arising from germline mutations in *RASA1* or *EPHB4*, with variable expressivity. Second hit somatic mutations are thought to account for the variable phenotypes (30, 31).

The skin lesions are multifocal pink or pale brown, round or ovoid, sometimes with a pale halo and telangiectatic features (Figure 17.16). Though these are referred to as CMs, they are high-flow lesions thought to represent micro arteriovenous fistulas (AVFs) (32). Approximately 30% of affected individuals have arteriovenous malformations (AVMs) or fistulae, which may involve any part of the body, including soft tissue, bone, spine, or brain (33, 34). Vein of Galen malformations of the brain have also been described. Intracranial or intraspinal high-flow lesions usually manifest in childhood or early adulthood (35).

Parkes Weber syndrome is the label given to a distinct phenotype of CM-AVM characterised by high-flow vascular anomalies (AVMs and AVFs) of the limb with overgrowth and has been described in the context of *RASA1* mutations and CM-AVM syndrome.

MRI/magnetic resonance angiography (MRA) of the head and MRI of the spine to look for central nervous system AVMs should be carried out at the time of diagnosis. Currently, there is no consensus

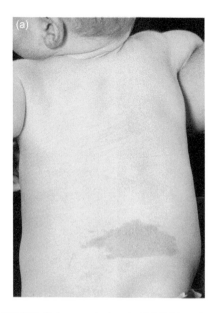
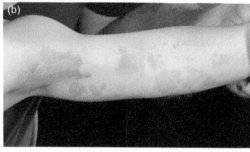

FIGURE 7.16 Cutaneous lesions in CM-AVM syndrome on (a) the lower back and (b) left medial upper arm in an 18-month-old male.

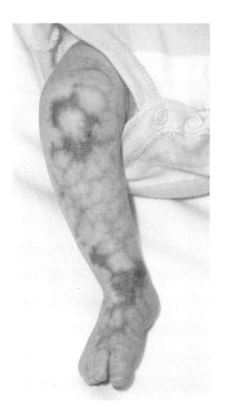

FIGURE 7.17 Cutis marmorata telangiectatica congenita of the right leg in a 9-week-old female.

on when further imaging should be carried out if the initial imaging is normal and if patients remain asymptomatic (35). However, re-scanning is required urgently if patients develop headaches or other neurological symptoms.

Clinical genetics input is required for clarification of the genetic status of at-risk relatives.

# CUTIS MARMORATA TELANGIECTATICA CONGENITA (CMTC)

Cutis marmorata telangiectatica congenita (CMTC) presents as a cutaneous dark red–purple reticulate vascular network associated with skin atrophy and sometimes ulceration (Figure 7.17). In most cases, it is localised and typically occurs in a segmental distribution. The vascular element does not resolve with warming, differentiating it from the physiological cutis marmorata frequently seen in newborns.

CMTC may be associated with limb asymmetry, including atrophy and leg length discrepancy. Glaucoma has been reported in cases of facial involvement by CMTC. In many cases, the vascular marks show improvement over time, but the atrophy tends to persist.

CMTC has been reported to arise from somatic mutations in *GNA11*.

Patients with CMTC on the face should be monitored for glaucoma and, when present on the lower limb, for leg length discrepancy (37–39).

---

### KEY MESSAGES

* The term capillary malformation is used for many different phenotypes.

* Some typical phenotypes will provide a clue to possible associated anomalies.

* A PWS-type CM of the forehead is associated with a risk of SWS and requires investigation with a brain MRI with contrast and prompt ophthalmology assessment.

* A CM involving the leg requires monitoring for leg length discrepancy.

---

- A diffuse CM with overgrowth must be distinguished from KTS.

- Monitoring of head circumference and neurodevelopment is required for infants with diffuse CM.

- Geographic CM is often associated with other segmental lymphatic and/or venous malformations.

- For infants presenting with multifocal CMs/telangiectatic lesions, consider CM-AVM syndrome and the need for imaging to look for central nervous system AVMs.

- Consider the potential psychosocial impact of visible differences arising from CMs and offer psychological support.

# REFERENCES

1. Kanada KN, Merin MR, Munden A, Friedlander SF. A prospective study of cutaneous findings in newborns in the United States: Correlation with race, ethnicity, and gestational status using updated classification and nomenclature. *J Pediatr*. 2012 Aug;161(2):240–5.
2. International Society for the Study of Vascular Anomalies. ISSVA Classification of Vascular Anomalies 2023. [Internet] [cited 2023]. Available from http://issva.org/classification
3. Rozas-Muñoz E, Frieden IJ, Roé E, Puig L, Baselga E. Vascular stains: Proposal for a clinical classification to improve diagnosis and management. *Pediatr Dermatol*. 2016;33(6):570–84.
4. Juern AM, Glick ZR, Drolet BA, Frieden IJ. Nevus simplex: A reconsideration of nomenclature, sites of involvement, and disease associations. *J Am Acad Dermatol*. 2010 Nov 1;63(5):805–14.
5. Guggisberg D, Hadj-Rabia S, Viney C, Bodemer C, Brunelle F, Zerah M, et al. Skin markers of occult spinal dysraphism in children: A review of 54 cases. *Arch Dermatol*. 2004 Sep 1;140(9):1109–15.
6. Klapman MH, Yao JF. Thickening and nodules in port-wine stains. *J Am Acad Dermatol*. 2001 Feb;44(2):300–2.
7. Prather HB, Arndt KA. The development of hypertrophy in port-wine stains, a common phenomenon that affects treatment recommendations. *Dermatol Surg Off Publ Am Soc Dermatol Surg Al*. 2015 Nov;41(11):1246–8.
8. Kim SJ, Kim YC. Eczema within a capillary malformation: A case of Meyerson phenomenon. *Ann Dermatol*. 2016 Dec;28(6):781–2.
9. Rancan A, Boscarelli A, Codrich D, Berti I, Guida E, Schleef J. Pyogenic granuloma arising within capillary malformations in children: A case report and literature review. *Dermatol Rep*. 2021 Aug 1;13(2):9115.
10. Shirley MD, Tang H, Gallione CJ, Baugher JD, Frelin LP, Cohen B, et al. Sturge-Weber syndrome and port-wine stains caused by somatic mutation in GNAQ. *N Engl J Med*. 2013 May 23;368(21):1971–9.
11. Higueros E, Roe E, Granell E, Baselga E. Sturge-Weber syndrome: A review. *Actas Dermosifiliogr*. 2017 Jun;108(5):407–17.
12. Waelchli R, Aylett SE, Robinson K, Chong WK, Martinez AE, Kinsler VA. New vascular classification of port-wine stains: Improving prediction of Sturge-Weber risk. *Br J Dermatol*. 2014 Oct;171(4):861–7.
13. Mantelli F, Bruscolini A, La Cava M, Abdolrahimzadeh S, Lambiase A. Ocular manifestations of Sturge-Weber syndrome: Pathogenesis, diagnosis, and management. *Clin Ophthalmol Auckl NZ*. 2016;10:871–8.
14. Sloneem J, Moss J, Powell S, Hawkins C, Fosi T, Richardson H, et al. The prevalence and profile of autism in Sturge-Weber syndrome. *J Autism Dev Disord*. 2022 May;52(5):1942–55.
15. Pinto ALR, Ou Y, Sahin M, Grant PE. Quantitative apparent diffusion coefficient mapping may predict seizure onset in children with Sturge-Weber syndrome. *Pediatr Neurol*. 2018 Jul;84:32–8.
16. Sabeti S, Ball KL, Bhattacharya SK, Bitrian E, Blieden LS, Brandt JD, et al. Consensus statement for the management and treatment of Sturge-Weber syndrome: Neurology, neuroimaging, and ophthalmology recommendations. *Pediatr Neurol*. 2021 Aug;121:59–66.
17. Zallmann M, Leventer RJ, Mackay MT, Ditchfield M, Bekhor PS, Su JC. Screening for Sturge-Weber syndrome: A state-of-the-art review. *Pediatr Dermatol*. 2018 Jan;35(1):30–42.
18. Huang L, Couto JA, Pinto A, Alexandrescu S, Madsen JR, Greene AK, et al. Somatic GNAQ mutation is enriched in brain endothelial cells in Sturge-Weber syndrome. *Pediatr Neurol*. 2017 Feb;67:59–63.
19. Wu Y, Peng C, Huang L, Xu L, Ding X, Liu Y, et al. Somatic GNAQ R183Q mutation is located within the sclera and episclera in patients with Sturge-Weber syndrome. *Br J Ophthalmol*. 2022 Jul;106(7):1006–11.
20. Sharan S, Swamy B, Taranath DA, Jamieson R, Yu T, Wargon O, et al. Port-wine vascular malformations and glaucoma risk in Sturge-Weber syndrome. *J AAPOS Off Publ Am Assoc Pediatr Ophthalmol Strabismus*. 2009 Aug;13(4):374–8.
21. Day AM, Hammill AM, Juhász C, Pinto AL, Roach ES, McCulloch CE, et al. Hypothesis: Presymptomatic treatment of Sturge-Weber syndrome with aspirin and antiepileptic drugs may delay seizure onset. *Pediatr Neurol*. 2019 Jan;90:8–12.
22. Bay MJ, Kossoff EH, Lehmann CU, Zabel TA, Comi AM. Survey of aspirin use in Sturge-Weber syndrome. *J Child Neurol*. 2011 Jun;26(6):692–702.
23. Thomas AC, Zeng Z, Rivière JB, O'Shaughnessy R, Al-Olabi L, St-Onge J, et al. Mosaic activating mutations in GNA11 and GNAQ are associated with phakomatosis pigmentovascularis and extensive dermal melanocytosis. *J Invest Dermatol*. 2016 Apr;136(4):770–8.
24. Goss JA, Konczyk DJ, Smits P, Sudduth CL, Bischoff J, Liang MG, et al. Diffuse capillary malformation with overgrowth contains somatic *PIK3CA* variants. *Clin Genet*. 2020 May;97(5):736–40.
25. Lee MS, Liang MG, Mulliken JB. Diffuse capillary malformation with overgrowth: A clinical subtype of vascular anomalies with hypertrophy. *J Am Acad Dermatol*. 2013 Oct;69(4):589–94.
26. Garde A, Guibaud L, Goldenberg A, Petit F, Dard R, Roume J, et al. Clinical and neuroimaging findings in 33 patients with MCAP syndrome: A survey to evaluate relevant endpoints for future clinical trials. *Clin Genet*. 2021 May;99(5):650–61.

27. Rivière JB, Mirzaa GM, O'Roak BJ, Beddaoui M, Alcantara D, Conway RL, et al. De novo germline and postzygotic mutations in *AKT3*, *PIK3R2* and *PIK3CA* cause a spectrum of related megalencephaly syndromes. *Nat Genet.* 2012 Jun 24;44(8):934–40.
28. Rodriguez-Laguna L, Ibañez K, Gordo G, Garcia-Minaur S, Santos-Simarro F, Agra N, et al. CLAPO syndrome: Identification of somatic activating *PIK3CA* mutations and delineation of the natural history and phenotype. *Genet Med Off J Am Coll Med Genet.* 2018 Aug;20(8):882–9.
29. Surveillance recommendations for children with overgrowth syndromes and predisposition to Wilms tumors and hepatoblastoma. PubMed [Internet]. [cited 2022 Dec 4]. Available from: https://pubmed.ncbi.nlm.nih.gov/28674120/
30. Macmurdo CF, Wooderchak-Donahue W, Bayrak-Toydemir P, Le J, Wallenstein MB, Milla C, et al. RASA1 somatic mutation and variable expressivity in capillary malformation/arteriovenous malformation (CM/AVM) syndrome. *Am J Med Genet A.* 2016 Jun;170(6):1450–4.
31. Lapinski PE, Doosti A, Salato V, North P, Burrows PE, King PD. Somatic second hit mutation of RASA1 in vascular endothelial cells in capillary malformation-arteriovenous malformation. *Eur J Med Genet.* 2018 Jan;61(1):11–6.
32. Valdivielso-Ramos M, Torrelo A, Martin-Santiago A, Hernández-Nuñez A, Azaña JM, Campos M, et al. Histopathological hallmarks of cutaneous lesions of capillary malformation-arteriovenous malformation syndrome. *J Eur Acad Dermatol Venereol JEADV.* 2020 Oct;34(10):2428–35.
33. Revencu N, Boon LM, Mendola A, Cordisco MR, Dubois J, Clapuyt P, et al. RASA1 mutations and associated phenotypes in 68 families with capillary malformation-arteriovenous malformation. *Hum Mutat.* 2013 Dec;34(12):1632–41.
34. Valdivielso-Ramos M, Martin-Santiago A, Azaña JM, Hernández-Nuñez A, Vera A, Perez B, et al. Capillary malformation-arteriovenous malformation syndrome: A multicentre study. *Clin Exp Dermatol.* 2021 Mar;46(2):300–5.
35. Orme CM, Boyden LM, Choate KA, Antaya RJ, King BA. Capillary malformation–arteriovenous malformation syndrome: Review of the literature, proposed diagnostic criteria, and recommendations for management. *Pediatr Dermatol.* 2013;30(4):409–15.
36. Iznardo H, Roé E, Puig L, Vikula M, López-Sánchez C, Baselga E. Good response to pulsed dye laser in patients with capillary malformation–arteriovenous malformation syndrome (CM-AVM). *Pediatr Dermatol.* 2020 Mar;37(2):342–4.
37. Tamburro J, Traboulsi EI, Patel MS. Isolated and classic cutis marmorata telangiectatica congenita. In: Adam MP, Everman DB, Mirzaa GM, Pagon RA, Wallace SE, Bean LJ, et al., editors. *GeneReviews®* [Internet]. Seattle (WA): University of Washington, Seattle; 1993 [cited 2022 Dec 1]. Available from: http://www.ncbi.nlm.nih.gov/books/NBK581081/
38. Bui TNPT, Corap A, Bygum A. Cutis marmorata telangiectatica congenita: A literature review. *Orphanet J Rare Dis.* 2019 Dec 4;14(1):283.
39. Haidari W, Light JG, Castellanos B, Jorizzo JL. Cutis marmorata telangiectasia congenita with painful ulcerations. *Dermatol Online J.* 2020 Jun 15;26(6):13030/qt1m99z767.

References

# Lymphatic Malformations

Sunit Davda and Richard J. Hewitt

## INTRODUCTION

Lymphatic malformations (LMs) encompass a spectrum of disorders, typically due to somatic mutations in the genes responsible for encoding oncogenic proliferation. They result in non-transportation of lymphatic fluid, lymphatic epithelial hyperplasia, or lymphatic obstruction. Whilst similar presentations can occur secondary to trauma or surgical disruption, the majority in clinical practice are congenital abnormalities which typically present in childhood.

Although not a new entity, with craniofacial LMs having been described in the 1800s, for example, variability in terminology has led to confusion around the topic with interchangeable use of terms leading to diagnostic uncertainty for clinicians, parents, and patients. The effect that LMs have on patients varies significantly from being relatively innocuous to carrying significant morbidity due to pain, infection, and mass effect.

Patients benefit from a multidisciplinary management approach, with treatments comprising a mixture of conservative management, medical treatments, image-guided intervention, and surgery, depending on the type of LM encountered and the needs of the child. More recently, focus has shifted to the potential of medical drug repurposing as causative gene mutations are identified, which has resulted in a rejuvenation of interest within this field and offers real hope for the future management of this condition.

## CLASSIFICATION

Over the years, there have been many names used interchangeably for this type of anomaly, which has contributed to significant confusion around this subject. The most commonly encountered historical terms include cystic hygroma (to describe cervicofacial LMs), lymphangioma, and lymphangiomatosis (a complex widespread lymphatic malformation). Terms such as these are obsolete and must be avoided.

According to the International Society for the Study of Vascular Anomalies (ISSVA) classification, LMs are vascular anomalies in which lymphatic fluid is predominant and are slow-flowing lesions (1). They fall into three main categories: common cystic, complex lymphatic anomalies (CLAs), and primary lymphoedema. CLAs are covered in Chapter 9.

Lymphoedema is caused by lymphatic dysfunction, leading to a localised interstitial accumulation of lymph fluid, with an increased risk of infection. Primary lymphoedema is a genetic developmental fault in either the function or structural make-up of the normal lymphatic conducting pathways. This is diagnosed and managed in an entirely different way to lymphatic anomalies, and although part of the classification, it is conceptually best considered a separate topic.

LMs can be associated with multiple other anomalies and tissue overgrowth, as part of the *PIK3CA*-related overgrowth spectrum (PROS). This includes complex and often poorly defined entities, such as Klippel–Trenaunay syndrome, CLOVES, CLAPO, and Proteus; these are covered in Chapters 7 and 12.

## COMMON CYSTIC LYMPHATIC MALFORMATIONS

The majority of LMs encountered in clinical practice fall under the term 'common cystic malformations', which consist of macrocystic lesions, microcystic lesions, or a combined type, and these three types are,

DOI: 10.1201/9781003257417-8

therefore, the focus of this chapter. Macrocystic LMs have been described as containing cysts greater than 1 cm in diameter, and microcystic as those containing cysts less than 1 cm. However, in practical terms, macrocysts can be best described as any cyst that can be individually visualised and measured by ultrasound, whereas microcysts are innumerable and not readily measurable, appearing as non-specific, spongiform, thickened tissue. Macrocystic lesions may consist of single unilocular cysts, but more commonly, they contain multiple cysts which can be interconnected. LMs tend to originate in the subcutaneous soft tissues but are typically trans-spatial anomalies, crossing fascial planes to involve a number of tissue types.

If an LM interferes with the main lymphatic channels, then lymphoedema can coexist, as lymph is now trapped within the tissues. These are called truncal LMs, as opposed to atruncal LMs (the more regularly encountered common cystic LM type), which are isolated anomalies with no connection to the main lymph drainage pathway.

# LYMPHATIC SYSTEM FUNCTION, DEVELOPMENT, AND GENETICS

The lymphatic system has three main roles (2). First, it has a role in regulation of fluid balance by resorption of fluid and solutes from the interstitial spaces of the body into the lymph vessels ultimately back to the blood circulation. Second, it is involved in transporting absorbed dietary fat from the gut as chylomicrons. Third, it is involved in immune priming within the lymph nodes. The lymphatic system has a passive function, i.e., driving interstitial fluid into the lymphatics through cyclical changes in oncotic and hydrostatic pressure, but also an active role in other processes, including gut absorption, movement of lymphocytes and antigen-presenting cells to the circulation, and regulating cerebrospinal fluid outflow.

Most of the lymph from the body and head and neck drains into the peripheral lymphatic vessels, which connect to larger trunks, eventually emptying into the centrally located thoracic duct (3). Lymph from the gut and lower half of the body drains into the cisterna chyli, which itself then drains into the thoracic duct. Only lymph from the right side of the head and neck, right thorax, and right upper limb drain into another structure – the right lymphatic duct. Both the thoracic duct and the right lymphatic duct drain into great veins of the neck to ensure lymphatic fluid returns to the venous circulation (Figure 8.1).

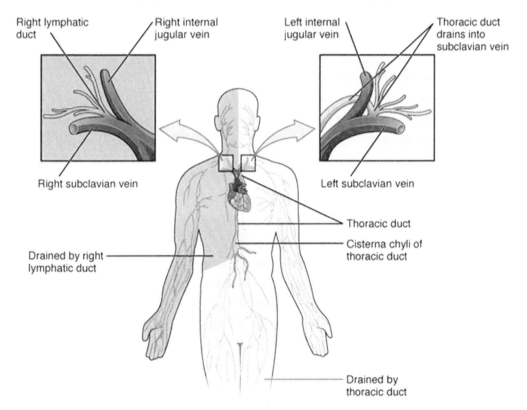

FIGURE 8.1 Pictorial representation of the lymphatic drainage routes of the body, depicting the areas of the body draining into the right lymphatic duct (purple) and the majority of the body draining into the thoracic duct (yellow).

The lymphatic system development starts at around Week 6. Lymphatic endothelial channels migrate out of embryonic veins, forming primitive lymphatic structures. After the primary lymphatic plexus has been established, it needs to mature into a hierarchical network of blind-ended capillaries, precollectors, and collecting vessels. The development of intraluminal (secondary) lymphatic valves in the collecting vessels ensures unidirectional flow of lymph through the system.

Impaired lymphatic function leads to accumulation of fluid in between cells in tissues, resulting in lymphedema, and mutations resulting in dysplastic or obstructed lymphatic vessels can result in chylothoraces, chylous ascites, or protein losing enteropathy. Meanwhile, lymphatic anomalies are due to abnormally formed lymphatic channels which are disconnected from the normal lymphatic drainage system.

LMs, like the CLAs, are caused by postzygotic somatic mutations in the RAS/MAPK and PI3K/AKT/mTOR pathways. The overall prevalence of LMs is 1 in every 4,000 live births (4). Common cystic LMs are most commonly due to somatic *PIK3CA* mutations, although mutations in *BRAF* and *PIK3R1* have also recently been described (5). The timing of the somatic mutation during fetal development determines the extent of the phenotype with more extensive LMs or LMs with associated overgrowth likely due to earlier mutations or a mutation affecting a progenitor cell with the capacity to differentiate into different cell types.

An appreciation of the underlying gene mutations has taken on greater significance due to repurposing of drug therapy that can target the mutation, especially in patients with complex phenotypes.

## HISTOLOGICAL APPEARANCE

LMs appear as thin-walled cystic lesions with a smooth surface on gross macroscopic inspection. Cut surface reveals the presence of macrocystic or microcystic disease, with large lymphatic channels in loose connective tissue stroma (Figure 8.2).

LMs are predominantly composed of abnormal, thin-walled channels lined by lymphatic-type bland endothelium. Normal tissues are infiltrated by a poorly circumscribed lesion composed of thin-walled lymphatic-type channels, which may show non-specific associated secondary changes. Within the background fibroadipose tissue, prominent lymphoid aggregates may be seen. The abnormal lymphatic-type vascular channels themselves often contain pale eosinophilic proteinaceous material with a minor population of macrophages and red blood cells.

Immunohistochemical staining confirms the lymphatic-type endothelium with expression of markers such as PROX1, VEGFR-3, CD37, CD34, D2-40 (podoplanin), and lymphatic vessel endothelial receptor 1 (LYVE-1). Electron microscopy will demonstrate poorly developed and discontinuous basal lamina and the presence of anchoring fibrils.

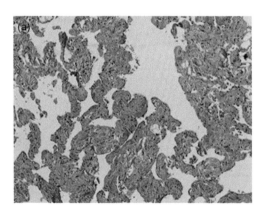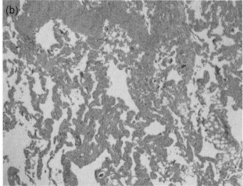

FIGURE 8.2 Photomicrographs: (a) original magnification x40, H&E, and (b) original magnification x100, H&E of a lymphatic malformation demonstrating a circumscribed and unencapsulated lesion composed of numerous thin-walled and irregularly shaped abnormal vascular channels, lined by a single layer of bland lymphatic type endothelium. The lymphatic endothelial nature can be confirmed by markers such as D2-40.

## CLINICAL PRESENTATION

LMs are present from birth and may remain clinically silent. They can present at any age, with, in recent years, more lesions being discovered prenatally with a rise in the incidence of fetal sonography

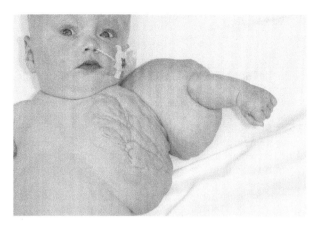

FIGURE 8.3 Lymphatic malformation in an infant affecting the left axilla, chest, and arm.

and magnetic resonance imaging (MRI). Postnatally, they often become clinically apparent during infancy or childhood (6). The exact presentation of LMs varies depending on location and type of lesion as well as the extent of a lesion, which can vary from a relatively tiny area to involve a whole limb (Figure 8.3). Typically, presentation is secondary to a degree of local mass effect, leading to a noticeable swelling from a subcutaneous lesion or compression or obstruction of nearby structures, for example, proptosis secondary to orbital involvement or respiratory distress and feeding difficulties from upper airway lesions.

LMs can involve any tissue within the body and are usually fairly localised. The skin and subcutaneous soft tissues are most commonly affected, but LMs can involve muscle, bone, and, more rarely, the visceral organs. When subcutaneous, they can present as soft compressible masses, similar to venous malformations (VMs), and may even have a blue hue (usually due to the presence of blood products in the cysts) but not to the same extent as VMs. On examination, LMs are usually soft and fluctuant, but they cannot be 'emptied' with compression, as they have no channels through which to drain, unlike VMs which can be emptied with compression or elevation and which re-fill with the help of gravity or increased venous pressure. This clinical sign is very helpful diagnostically in differentiating between the two slow-flow malformation subtypes.

Overall, LMs usually grow slowly at the same rate as the patient, though occasionally they demonstrate spontaneous involution, especially in the first few months of life. Events such as intralesional bleeding or a concurrent infection can cause lesions to rapidly expand, but this is usually temporary. Increased swelling at the time of a concurrent illness is, diagnostically, a very helpful feature of the history of an LM; the endothelial lining of the cysts produces more fluid at the same time as the body's lymphatic system when it responds to an inflammatory process. Note that the cysts are not in direct communication with the lymphatic system but are acting in tandem with it. Intralesional bleeds can be painful due to the sudden expansion of the cysts. This process does not signal any venous or arterial component to the malformation; it is simply a leak from a normal vessel in the fragile walls of the cysts – a leak which continues until the pressure within the cyst causes tamponade. This process can lead to repeated episodes of bruising, which can be distressing for the child and the caregiver.

Infection is an unusual presentation amongst the vascular anomalies. Patients may present with cellulitis, secondary abscess formation of an infected macrocyst, or even systemic illness, requiring antibiotics and occasionally hospital admission.

Microcystic disease, when it involves the skin or mucosal surface, can appear as raised tiny vesicles, which can be white, red, blue, or black in colour. They may weep serous or serosanguinous fluid and can bleed. Such microcystic vesicles can be found on any area of skin or mucous membrane and are often found in the oral cavity, feet, or perineum.

When LMs are multifocal or are present alongside another abnormality, such as bone cyst lesions, chylous effusions (pleural, pericardial, peritoneal), or protein-losing abnormalities, then one of the CLAs (e.g., Gorham–Stout disease [GSD], generalized lymphatic anomaly [GLA], central conducting lymphatic anomaly [CCLA], etc.) should be suspected (see Chapter 9).

In the majority of patients, LMs are caused by somatic mutations. Risk factors include trisomy 21, Turner syndrome, and children of older mothers; however, the vast majority of patients do not fall within one of these categories.

# REGIONS OF INVOLVEMENT

### HEAD AND NECK

LMs are most common in the head and neck, comprising 75% of lesions encountered. Lesions of the head and neck pose unique challenges, as they are often trans-spatial, and surgical resection is often not possible due to the risks of nerve injury, soft tissue deformity, and functional impairment. Microcystic malformations, in particular, present surgical challenges due to their infiltrative nature and lack of clear margins. LMs involving the airway tend to be above the true vocal folds. The most common is oral cavity involvement, but they can also involve the oropharynx and hypopharynx as well as parapharyngeal or retropharyngeal lesions. Involvement of the glottis, subglottis, and trachea is rare. Salivary gland involvement can occur, and the parotid gland is the most common site of involvement (7, 8).

LMs in the tongue tend to be poorly defined, diffuse, microcystic lesions. There is often a characteristic vesicular appearance to the lingual surface; the tiny vesicles turn from pink to black with inflammation of the malformation, such as with spicy foods, and can be painful. Cross sectional imaging is often required to determine the true extent of deep extension and plan treatment. Children often present with recurrent episodes of enlargement, and the macroglossia can lead to airway obstruction, swallowing difficulties, speech disturbance, excessive salivation, and malocclusion.

LMs in the neck can be classified as Stage I (unilateral infrahyoid), Stage II (unilateral suprahyoid), Stage III (unilateral suprahyoid and infrahyoid), Stage IV (bilateral suprahyoid), Stage V (bilateral suprahyoid and infrahyoid), and Stage VI (bilateral infrahyoid). This staging may help in determining the risk of complications and surgical outcomes (9).

### CUTANEOUS AND MUCOSAL DISEASE

Cutaneous LMs, known as lymphangioma circumscriptum, are hyperkeratotic papules which often lead to skin vesicles containing clear fluid or blood (Figure 8.4). Similar lesions can occur in mucosal surfaces such as the buccal mucosa or palate. These foci are prone to ulceration, secondary infection, and haemorrhage. The most frequent sites of involvement are the proximal extremities, trunk, axilla, and the oral cavity.

### MUSCULOSKELETAL

LMs of the extremities are common and are almost always confined to the subcutaneous fat. Cystic disease originating from the muscle compartments is rare and should prompt consideration of alternative diagnoses. When there is associated overgrowth of a limb, PROS should be considered.

Intraosseous lesions are typically part of more CLAs; when one lesion is identified, a low threshold is advised for screening for multiple lesions, given the multifocal nature of many CLAs.

### THORACIC

LMs in the axillary region are the second most common site of disease following the head and neck. LMs may be found in the mediastinum, the lung and pleura, and the pericardium. As with other locations, these can be trans-spatial, involving multiple tissue types. Diffuse lesions may leak chylous or non-chylous fluid into the pericardium or pleural spaces, which can be extremely challenging to manage.

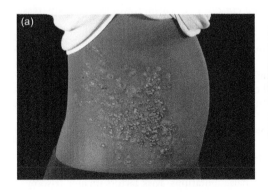
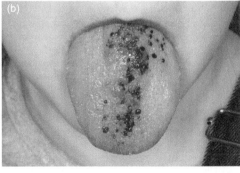

FIGURE 8.4 Examples of superficial lymphatic malformations affecting (a) the skin (also known as lymphangioma circumscriptum) and (b) the mucosa of the tongue.

Lymphatic Malformations

Occult mediastinal lesions are often contiguous with lesions of the neck or thoracic inlet and, thus, are often detected when cross sectional imaging of the craniofacial region is performed. As such, the upper mediastinum should be included in any neck imaging. Larger lesions resulting in respiratory compromise require intervention, but small traces of disease in the mediastinum are rarely of significance.

## ABDOMINAL

Visceral involvement is rare. Splenic lesions are usually subcapsular but can be intraparenchymal. The differential diagnosis of these includes benign splenic or hydatid cysts.

Abdominal LMs make up 5% of presentations, with the most common site being mesenteric or retroperitoneal (10). These tend to be occult but can present with loss of appetite, failure to thrive, haemorrhage, volvulus, obstruction, and, rarely, bowel ischaemia due to compression or volvulus. In the abdomen, they are more commonly macrocystic. Involvement of the small bowel mesentery is more common than the large bowel. These can be imaged with ultrasound, MRI, or computed tomography (CT) (Figure 8.5). The main differentials are enteric duplication cysts, pseudocysts, and teratoma. Involvement of the bowel itself is rare and is usually discovered incidentally during endoscopy. When the bowel is involved, protein-losing enteropathy may be encountered.

## UROGENITAL

LMs rarely involve the upper urinary tract. Urinary bladder or urethral involvement often results in intermittent but persistent episodes of haematuria, usually requiring cystoscopy for confirmation of the diagnosis and assessment of the extent of the disease. Urothelial involvement looks very similar to the mucosal involvement described above.

Scrotal LMs are also uncommon lesions. When they occur, the scrotal wall or tunics are most often involved, with testicular, epididymal, or spermatic cord involvement being less commonly involved. Most will present as painless swelling, but given the rarity, it is not uncommon for these to be misdiagnosed as a complex hydrocoele or haematocoele. Recurrence of a hydrocoele after surgical intervention should prompt consideration of this diagnosis. In female patients, ovarian and uterine involvement is very rare. Involvement of the vulva and surrounding tissues is more common, and as these lesions grow with age, they may become clinically more evident as the external genitalia develop. The size and location of these lesions can carry significant psychosocial concerns as children progress into adolescence. Multidisciplinary input and psychology services involvement are often required. Patients with superficial vesicles may leak fluid, and this can also be difficult to manage.

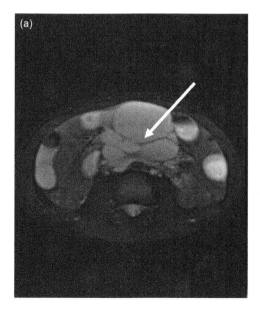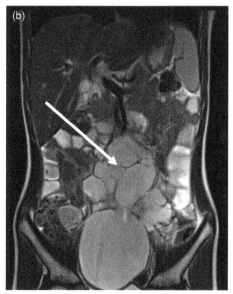

FIGURE 8.5 (a) Axial and (b) coronal T2-weighted fat-suppressed MRI images in a child presenting with abdominal distention, demonstrating multiple high-signal intensity cysts within the mesentery (arrows) in keeping with a mesenteric lymphatic malformation.

# IMAGING

## FETAL IMAGING

Advances in fetal sonographic techniques and the increasing adoption of fetal MRI has led to better evaluation of these LMs, in particular, large craniofacial LMs. There has also been increased early recognition of these lesions, as more women have imaging later in pregnancy for other reasons; these lesions seem to grow later than the usual anatomical anomaly scan, which occurs at around 20 weeks gestation. Fetal MRI is best used as a complementary examination for large lesions initially identified on ultrasound, for further evaluation of the extent of the malformation, in particular when detailed management plans regarding delivery and early postnatal care are required (Figure 8.6). These imaging modalities also play a significant role in parental counselling.

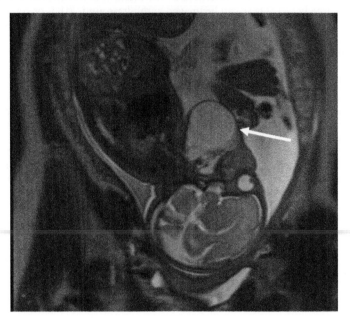

FIGURE 8.6 Sagittal T2-weighted fetal MRI image demonstrating a craniofacial lymphatic malformation with a thin-walled high signal intensity (bright) macrocystic component (arrow) in the anterior neck of the fetus.

## ULTRASOUND

The mainstay of diagnostic imaging for LMs is ultrasound (11). On ultrasound, macrocystic lesions appear as unilocular or multilocular cysts. They may have internal septa of varying thickness. Typically, the fluid within the cysts is anechoic, but there may be low level echoes or debris from proteinaceous content within it due to prior haemorrhage or infection. Colour Doppler is useful to confirm the absence of flow within the cysts, though there may be some flow detected, of course, from normal stromal vessels within the septae or surrounding parenchyma. Typically, the cysts are thin-walled, but if there has been infection or recent sclerotherapy, a thicker rind may be seen. Microcystic disease looks more like heterogenous echogenic solid tissue with tiny anechoic foci within it (Figure 8.7). Most notably, the tissues will be considerably denser compared to the surrounding soft tissues. Note that microcystic disease tends to be associated with a generalised increase in the volume of subcutaneous fat immediately surrounding it, and the fat can be of a different echotexture to the normal soft tissues. This is important to appreciate when it comes to predicting response to sclerotherapy, as the cysts may shrink, but the bulky fat will persist.

Ultrasound is a particularly useful tool in the outpatient clinic. It allows the interventional radiologist to confirm the diagnosis, provide a visual demonstration of the lesion for the child and guardians, and assess potential targets for treatment. Ultrasound may, however, underestimate the extent and depth of larger or more complex lesions, and this is where cross sectional imaging is useful.

## MRI

The next most commonly used imaging investigation is MRI due to its improved soft tissue resolution, lack of ionising radiation (important in young children with particularly radiosensitive tissues), and

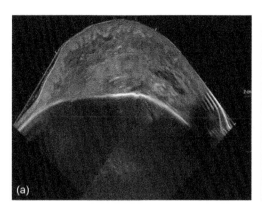
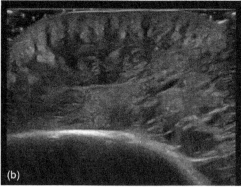

FIGURE 8.7 Ultrasound study of a subcutaneous microcystic lymphatic malformation of the forehead, with (a) an extended field-of-view image giving an overview of the size and complexity of the lesion, and (b) a detailed image of the malformation highlighting the markedly heterogenous soft tissue and the dark or hypoechoic slit-like fluid filled spaces at the centre of the lesion.

ability to identify the depth and extent of the malformation (for example, into the deep spaces of the neck, mediastinum, or other vital structures). MRI is useful in patients for which ultrasound may only identify the 'tip of the iceberg' (Figure 8.8); however, in young children it usually necessitates the use of general anaesthesia, so judicious use of this investigation in the early years is required.

Lesions that have not been complicated by infection or haemorrhage are typically bright (hyperintense) on T2-weighted sequences and dark (hypointense) on T1-weighted sequences; the T1 signal can be variable if proteinaceous content is present from haemorrhage or infection. Haemorrhage can also give the appearance of fluid/fluid levels (Figure 8.9); however, this imaging feature is not pathognomonic, as it is also seen from the settling out of stagnant blood in VMs. Postcontrast imaging

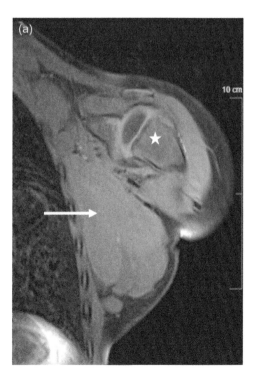
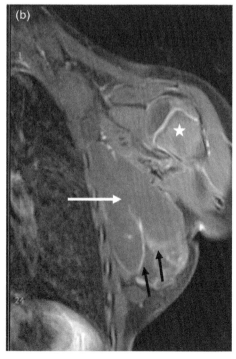

Imaging

FIGURE 8.8 Coronal T1-weighted fat-suppressed MRI images of a macrocystic lymphatic malformation in the left axilla of a teenager (white arrow). The asterisk denotes the left humeral head. (a) Without contrast enhancement, the lesion is poorly differentiated from the surrounding soft tissues; (b) postcontrast administration, there is characteristic enhancement of the walls and septae of the lesion (black arrows) but no central enhancement.

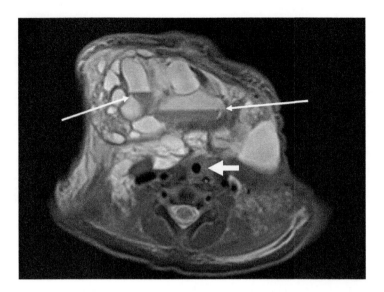

FIGURE 8.9 Axial T2-weighted fat-supressed MRI image of an infant with a complex lymphatic malformation involving multiple fascial planes and spaces in the neck. The high signal (bright) malformation contains both macrocystic and microcystic or more solid components. The central macrocysts contain fluid-fluid levels (long white arrows) of differing signal intensity, reflecting blood layering in the cysts from a previous intralesional haemorrhage. Note that the trachea (short white arrow) is slightly deviated to the left by the malformation.

demonstrates enhancement of the walls but, importantly, no enhancement of the cyst contents, which differentiates it from a VM. Microcystic disease, which consists of spongiform, rather than solid disease, often demonstrates diffuse, ill-defined hyperintense T2 signal and hypointense T1 signal on MRI, with diffuse, mild stromal enhancement.

## CT

CT rarely gives any more information than ultrasound or MRI. LMs will appear as homogenous cystic lesions on CT or may demonstrate some heterogeneity if there is blood or proteinaceous material within the lesion. The lesions may be simple or may show thin internal septations. Given the radiation burden associated with CT, it should be reserved for those situations in which MRI is not readily available but when anatomic localisation and definition of lesions is urgently required, for example in an acute setting. It should always be followed up with ultrasound and/or MRI imaging.

### WHICH IMAGING TEST TO CHOOSE?

Ultrasound is typically the first imaging modality of choice. It is a useful tool for clinic settings, providing adequate diagnostic information for superficial lesions. There is no ionising radiation or need for sedation. Recent guidelines from the Vascular Anomalies Working Group of the European Reference Network on Rare Multisystemic Vascular Diseases (VASCERN) also recommend the routine use of MRI prior to any sclerotherapy or surgical intervention (12). In situations in which there is concern over involvement of vital structures, e.g., craniofacial malformations, or prior to complicated surgical or sclerotherapy planning, MRI should be considered essential. However, in other cases, such as focal extremity lesions with a characteristic history, examination, and ultrasound findings, the treatment can often be initiated without the need for MRI.

## BIOPSY

Obtaining tissue for histological and genetic evaluation may be useful in some cases to confirm the type of vascular anomaly but also to search for underlying somatic mutations, which are present only in affected tissue. However, this is rarely used in common cystic LMs and would only be advisable in atypical cases with diagnostic uncertainty, following discussion in a multidisciplinary setting. If advances in medical therapeutic options continue, there may be an increased role for biopsy in the future.

# THERAPEUTIC OPTIONS

The therapeutic options depend on the location and size of the malformation, the affected tissue, the experience of the physicians, and above all, the clinical status of the patient. Many children may be asymptomatic, and the risks of intervention may far outweigh the risks of watchful waiting.

## CONSERVATIVE

The clinical management of any LM should be centred on the child's clinical symptoms and take into account the wishes of the child and guardians, when possible. It is important to help the family to understand that the malformation is part of the way the child's body is made and can almost never be completely removed. This message often bears repeating. LMs can fluctuate in size with concurrent illnesses or intralesional haemorrhage, a common cause of repeated episodes of painful swelling and bruising which may prompt intervention. Infections are less common but can be difficult to manage if they occur. But many children may never be significantly troubled by their LM, and it may be possible to watch and wait without intervention. As children grow older, malformations that are clearly visible may be linked to insecurities about their differences in appearance; close involvement with psychology services can be extremely beneficial (see Chapter 4). Compression garments usually have no role in the management of LMs.

## MEDICAL THERAPY

Sirolimus, an mTOR inhibitor, is used in the treatment of symptomatic LMs not amenable to sclerotherapy or surgery. Sirolimus may reduce the volume of the lesion and decrease pain as well as possibly improve the mucosal and skin infiltration effects of LMs (13). Decision-making around the instigation of medical therapy, as well as the administration and maintenance of the therapy, is usually overseen by dermatologists or haematologists with expertise in vascular anomalies. Recent data has also shown alpelisib, a specific inhibitor of PI3K-alpha, may have a role in the treatment of LMs refractory to sirolimus, although further evidence is required to determine its safety and efficacy in a larger cohort of patients.

## PERCUTANEOUS SCLEROTHERAPY

Image-guided sclerotherapy is often the first-line intervention for LMs. Simple aspiration of a cyst will only result in recurrence of the swelling, as the active cyst lining will continue to produce lymphatic fluid. The use of sclerosants for controlled destruction of the cyst itself has been used for many years (14). In LMs, surgical cure is often very difficult to achieve in practice, and the alternative of minimally invasive sclerotherapy is often preferred, especially for macrocystic LMs. Advantages include no surgical scars, reduced risk of neurovascular injury, and quick recovery times. Repeated treatments are often required, and there is a significant risk of recurrence over the longer term; however, the procedures are usually well tolerated by patients. It is important to explore the family's expectations around treatment outcomes prior to embarking on a sclerotherapy program. Sclerotherapy should always be promoted as a means of symptom control rather than a cure. Most children and guardians want the malformation to disappear, which is entirely understandable, and may struggle to maintain more realistic expectations. This is why it is important for interventional radiologists to be part of the clinical team and ensure they have these conversations regularly with the family in an outpatient setting.

Sclerosant agents used in LMs include sodium tetradecyl sulfate (STS), doxycycline, polidocanol, dehydrated alcohol, and bleomycin. In some countries, OK432 is available, which also produces good results. The various sclerosant agents have different mechanisms of action (15). STS, polidocanol, and dehydrated alcohol induce immediate injury of the cyst walls leading to irritation of the cysts, apposition of the cyst walls, and eventual scarring of the malformation. The main action of agents such as doxycycline and OK432 is to induce a low-grade inflammatory process at the centre of the malformation, with similar results. Bleomycin is a cytotoxic agent; it causes DNA degradation in solid tissue. Its mechanism of action when used as a sclerosing agent is poorly understood, but it makes sense that it is likely to be more effective in 'solid' microcystic disease.

The risks of sclerotherapy vary according to the agent used but include skin ulceration, scarring and necrosis, secondary infection, nerve damage, and non-target sclerotherapy effects. However, each sclerosant also has its own unique side effects to be aware of. For example, doxycycline carries a potential risk of haemolytic anaemia and metabolic acidosis in neonates. With bleomycin, operators and anaesthetists should be aware of the risks of long-term skin hyperpigmentation following localised skin trauma, hypersensitivity-type reactions, and the theoretical risk of pulmonary fibrosis following systemic bleomycin exposure; standardised precautions should be taken to minimise these risks. In addition, accurate

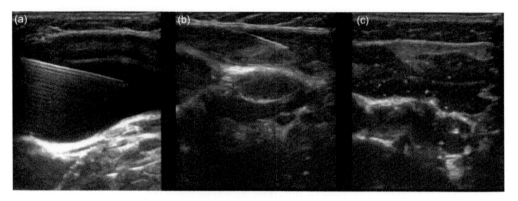

FIGURE 8.10 Series of three ultrasound images demonstrating (a) the needle going into a cyst, (b) the reduction in the size of the cyst following fluid aspiration, and (c) then instillation of sclerosant into the cyst as demonstrated by the cyst becoming distended again and now containing low level echoes from the instilled drug.

dose documentation for bleomycin is important, given the risk of systemic toxicity with cumulative dosing and recommendations around cumulative lifetime dose limits (usually taken to be 2,000–3,000 IU/kg in children and 80,000–100,000 IU in adults). Operators should be aware of the various units used to define bleomycin dose in different countries and in the scientific literature so that inadvertent dose errors are not made (see Chapter 10).

The procedural approach for sclerotherapy may vary with operator preference; however, the general principles are the same (Figure 8.10). Procedures are generally performed as day cases under general anaesthetic in a sterile environment. Under ultrasound guidance, 20–23G needles or peripheral cannulas are used to access the lesion percutaneously. As much fluid as possible is aspirated to ensure that the sclerosing agent is not diluted unnecessarily and that the cysts are not overdistended when sclerosant is instilled. The fluid is usually serous, serosanguinous, or brown (from altered blood), but can be chylous in truncal lesions. Intralesional needle tip position may be confirmed with contrast and fluoroscopic guidance if required (Figure 8.11). Once the fluid has been aspirated, sclerosant is instilled under continuous ultrasound guidance to assess cyst distension and minimise the risk that non-target areas receive sclerosant. Ultrasound will demonstrate low level echoes from the sclerosant fluid within the cyst as well as allow for communicating cysts to be identified as the sclerosant percolates through the lesion. Being careful not to over distend the cysts, the sclerosant is then left *in situ* to act.

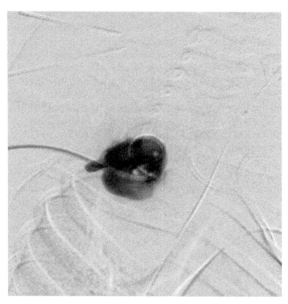

FIGURE 8.11 Digitally subtracted radiographic image of a child with a lymphatic malformation of the neck, showing the pigtail drain in a right supraclavicular cyst. Radiopaque contrast medium has been administered through the drain to confirm its position within the cyst.

Larger cysts may benefit from temporary percutaneous drain placement and serial sclerotherapy procedures over several days. Once most of the fluid has been aspirated via one or more small drains placed into the largest cysts, the sclerosant can be instilled into the cyst cavity through the drain(s). The drains are then left *in situ* for serial sclerotherapy procedures over 24–72 hours. Most children will tolerate these repeat sclerotherapy procedures via the drain awake, with local anaesthesia instilled into the lesion through the drain approximately 10 minutes prior to instillation of sclerosant. The drain is typically left closed for 2–6 hours after each procedure while the drug acts and then opened for up to 24 hours for the resultant reactive fluid collection to drain.

The usual drug of choice for sclerotherapy in macrocystic lesions, due to a combination of its safety profile, tolerance, availability, effectiveness, and cost, is doxycycline, though sodium tetradecyl sulfate, polidocanol, and dehydrated alcohol, amongst others, are also popular. Larger cysts, in particular, may benefit from 'pretreatment' with STS, which is instilled, left to dwell for 5–10 minutes, and then withdrawn prior to instillation of doxycycline in an attempt to achieve improved outcomes. The theory behind this is that STS denatures the cyst's endothelium, increasing the membrane permeability to doxycycline.

Sclerotherapy of macrocystic lesions usually causes inflammation and swelling of the malformation for 1–2 weeks. The degree of swelling and discomfort is usually related to the agent used and proportional to the dose instilled, although reaction to the treatment can be remarkably variable. Bleomycin causes the least swelling of any agents, so it should be the agent of choice in sites highly sensitive to swelling, such as the retro-orbit or carpal tunnel. Response to treatment is generally seen as a slow process over the next 2–3 months. Malformations of any great size or consisting of multiple macrocysts will almost certainly need more than one treatment; many operators choose to book a series of procedures, each a few weeks apart, before pausing to assess for response.

Microcystic LMs are most commonly treated with bleomycin, with infiltration of the sclerosant throughout the microcystic tissue, aiming to reduce overall lesion bulk. Note, however, that the surrounding fatty overgrowth tends to persist.

## LASER AND ABLATIVE THERAPIES

Laser ablation can be used to reduce oozing from superficial dermal or mucosal lymphatic vesicles and to improve the cosmetic appearance of the skin. Different techniques exist, such as carbon dioxide laser, which are useful in cutaneous lesions. For oral cavity lesions, yttrium aluminium garnet (NdYAG) laser is particularly effective. Pulsed dye laser can be used but has limited penetration, and, thus, its use is likely limited to cutaneous malformations. Coblation (a word derived from 'controlled ablation') is now commonly used for ENT and arthroscopic procedures. It involves using low-temperature radiofrequency and a saline solution to gently and precisely remove layers of tissue. Although it is not a permanent solution, it is remarkably effective at removing the lymphatic vesicles of tongue LMs and allowing the tongue to re-surface with more normal tissue. It can be repeated at intervals to keep painful or bleeding microcystic mucosal disease under control.

Minimally invasive therapies such as radiofrequency ablation (RF), cryoablation, and reversible electroporation have been used more recently and are showing some benefit in selected cases where standard therapies have failed.

## SURGICAL TECHNIQUES

Surgery for LMs is very challenging in all cases except superficial macrocystic lesions (Figure 8.12). Complex mixed macro- and microcystic lesions are often intimately related to major blood vessels, nerves, and musculature as well as close to vital structures, particularly in the head and neck. Surgery for these cases is usually reserved for residual small, scarred lesions postsclerotherapy in which operative morbidity is much lower and the option for cosmetic intervention to address excess redundant skin or asymmetry can be undertaken simultaneously. Functional outcome is clearly a key aim of treatment. In some lesions, such as the tongue, debulking of the lesion may give a better functional outcome than repeated sclerotherapy.

Newer surgical techniques can offer help in managing the morbidity of small unresectable lesions. For example, mucosal excoriation, bleeding, and pain is often associated with lesions abutting/involving the oral cavity, and these can be treated with coblation to resurface mucosal areas where conservative measures are insufficient.

More major surgical interventions need to be meticulously planned and undertaken with a multidisciplinary team, highlighting the risks involved with major surgery such as acute blood loss, postoperative seroma formation, infection, contractures, and poor wound healing (16) (Figure 8.13). Occupational therapists and physiotherapists lend significant value in terms of controlling postoperative swelling with compression garments and managing functional rehabilitation. There may be a role for sclerotherapy of the resection cavity postoperatively in instances of seroma formation.

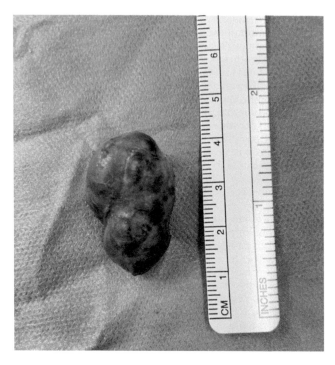

FIGURE 8.12 Surgically excised macrocystic lymphatic malformation of the neck.

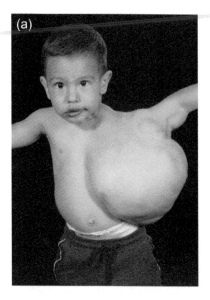
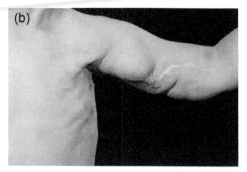

FIGURE 8.13 A young child with a very large lymphatic malformation of the left chest wall, (a) before and (b) after surgical resection.

## EXIT PROCEDURE AND AIRWAY MANAGEMENT

The antenatal diagnosis of an LM affecting the head and neck of a fetus usually leads to clinical concern. *Ex utero* intrapartum treatment (EXIT) is a technique to secure the fetal airway while perinatal oxygenation is maintained through the utero-placental circulation. EXIT procedures are performed under planned maternal general anaesthetic (17). Following uterine incision, strict haemostatic control from the incision is required due to the risk of torrential haemorrhage from uterine contractions. The fetus is partially delivered whilst remaining connected to the maternal placental circulation, the airway secured by an experienced paediatric anaesthetic and ENT team (via intubation or occasionally tracheostomy), oxytocin is administered, and the fetus delivered. Once stabilised, the neonate is re-imaged and a management strategy discussed which may involve early planned sclerotherapy or surgical debulking. Often the child is more stable than predicted antenatally, and intervention can be delayed until multidisciplinary discussions have been had and the family counselled as to the prognosis and various treatment options available. When possible, intervention should be deferred until strictly necessary. In babies for whom the airway is severely compromised, tracheostomy can be necessary whilst regular procedures such as sclerotherapy (percutaneous or transoral) or surgical debulking continue. The expectation is usually that the tracheostomy will not be required for more than a few years, though these cases can be extremely challenging and long-term tracheostomy is required by a small subset of children.

## INTRA-ABDOMINAL LYMPHATIC DISEASE

LMs can occur within the root of the mesentery and in the retroperitoneum. The symptoms are often non-specific, with children presenting with abdominal distention, non-specific abdominal pain, or loss of appetite. They can be a diagnostic challenge; teratoma should always be considered in the differential. Surgical excision of the most extensive of these lesions can require the removal of a significant portion of bowel. Sclerotherapy can be performed percutaneously, usually with a slow but excellent response. Occasionally, the subsequent inflammation and irritation of bowel leads to a temporary ileus. Combined assessment and intervention by a surgeon and interventional radiologist is often a pragmatic approach for mesenteric lesions, allowing laparoscopic assessment of the lesion before any final decision is made regarding surgical resection or sclerotherapy. A percutaneous drain can be placed into the macrocystic components followed by drainage of the cyst. Under laparoscopic vision, the origin of the malformation can then be assessed for the feasibility of laparoscopic resection, based on how broad the attachment is. If it is felt that complete resection would be technically challenging or too radical an intervention, sclerotherapy can then be performed through the drain.

---

### KEY MESSAGES

- LMs are a spectrum of disorders, of which simple cystic LMs are most likely to be encountered in clinical practice. These are further subdivided into macrocystic, microcystic, and mixed.

- These are postzygotic somatic mutations, typically involving the *PIK3CA* pathway, with a prevalence of 1 in 4,000 live births.

- Distribution can vary, and it can affect almost every part of the body, often become clinically apparent during infancy or childhood, with presentations varying depending on location of lesion. Most commonly they affect the head and neck.

- Patients often present following intralesional bleeding or concurrent infection which causes rapid growth in lesions. Microcytic disease may involve skin or mucous membranes.

- Ultrasound is the first-line imaging investigation of choice, often used in clinic to help diagnose the lesion and formulate a management plan. MRI is useful for determining the full extent of the lesion and whether it affects vital structures; however, it often requires a general anaesthetic.

- Treatment options can vary and require multidisciplinary decision-making. When indicated, image-guided percutaneous sclerotherapy and surgery, sometimes in combination, are the mainstay of treatment. Medical management, through drug repurposing, as genetic pathways are elucidated shows promise for the future.

---

# REFERENCES

1. International Society for the Study of Vascular Anomalies. ISSVA Classification of Vascular Anomalies 2023. [Internet] [cited 2023]. Available from http://issva.org/classification
2. Breslin JW, Yang Y, Scallan JP, Sweat RS, Adderley SP, Murfee WL. Lymphatic vessel network structure and physiology. *Compr Physiol*. 2018 Dec 13;9(1):207–99.

3. Null M, Agarwal M. Anatomy, lymphatic system. In: *StatPearls* [Internet]. Treasure Island (FL): StatPearls Publishing; 2022 [cited 2022 Dec 18]. Available from: http://www.ncbi.nlm.nih.gov/books/NBK513247/

4. Gallagher JR, Martini J, Carroll S, Small A, Teng J. Annual prevalence estimation of lymphatic malformation with a cutaneous component: Observational study of a national representative sample of physicians. *Orphanet J Rare Dis*. 2022 Dec;17(1):192.

5. Mäkinen T, Boon LM, Vikkula M, Alitalo K. Lymphatic malformations: Genetics, mechanisms and therapeutic strategies. *Circ Res*. 2021 Jun 25;129(1):136–54.

6. Kronfli AP, McLaughlin CJ, Moroco AE, Grant CN. Lymphatic malformations: A 20-year single institution experience. *Pediatr Surg Int*. 2021 Jun;37(6):783–90.

7. Adams MT, Saltzman B, Perkins JA. Head and neck lymphatic malformation treatment: A systematic review. *Otolaryngol Neck Surg*. 2012 Oct;147(4):627–39.

8. Lerat J, Mounayer C, Scomparin A, Orsel S, Bessede JP, Aubry K. Head and neck lymphatic malformation and treatment: Clinical study of 23 cases. *Eur Ann Otorhinolaryngol Head Neck Dis*. 2016 Dec;133(6):393–6.

9. Hamoir M, Plouin-Gaudon I, Rombaux P, Francois G, Cornu AS, Desuter G, et al. Lymphatic malformations of the head and neck: A retrospective review and a support for staging. *Head Neck*. 2001 Apr;23(4):326–37.

10. Francavilla ML, White CL, Oliveri B, Lee EY, Restrepo R. Intraabdominal lymphatic malformations: Pearls and pitfalls of diagnosis and differential diagnoses in pediatric patients. *Am J Roentgenol*. 2017 Mar;208(3):637–49.

11. Snyder EJ, Sarma A, Borst AJ, Tekes A. Lymphatic anomalies in children: Update on imaging diagnosis, genetics, and treatment. *Am J Roentgenol*. 2022 Jun;218(6):1089–101.

12. Ghaffarpour N, Baselga E, Boon LM, Diociaiuti A, Dompmartin A, Dvorakova V, et al. The VASCERN-VASCA working group diagnostic and management pathways for lymphatic malformations. *Eur J Med Genet*. 2022 Dec;65(12):104637.

13. Wiegand S, Dietz A, Wichmann G. Efficacy of sirolimus in children with lymphatic malformations of the head and neck. *Eur Arch Oto-Rhino-Laryngol Off J Eur Fed Oto-Rhino-Laryngol Soc EUFOS Affil Ger Soc Oto-Rhino-Laryngol – Head Neck Surg*. 2022 Aug;279(8):3801–10.

14. Balakrishnan K, Menezes MD, Chen BS, Magit AE, Perkins JA. Primary surgery vs primary sclerotherapy for head and neck lymphatic malformations. *JAMA Otolaryngol Neck Surg*. 2014 Jan 1;140(1):41.

15. Albanese G, Kondo KL. Pharmacology of sclerotherapy. *Semin Interv Radiol*. 2010 Dec;27(4):391–9.

16. Bajaj Y, Hewitt R, Ifeacho S, Hartley BEJ. Surgical excision as primary treatment modality for extensive cervicofacial lymphatic malformations in children. *Int J Pediatr Otorhinolaryngol*. 2011 May;75(5):673–7.

17. Butler CR, Maughan EF, Pandya P, Hewitt R. Ex utero intrapartum treatment (EXIT) for upper airway obstruction. *Curr Opin Otolaryngol Head Neck Surg*. 2017 Apr;25(2):119–26.

# 9 Complex Lymphatic Anomalies

Mary Glover, Maanasa Polubothu, Sunit Davda, and Premal A. Patel

## INTRODUCTION

The lymphatic system comprises a unidirectional hierarchal vascular system, the main role of which is to enable fluid homeostasis by absorbing extravasated fluid from the blood vascular system. In a healthy adult, at least three litres of fluid are absorbed daily from peripheral tissues and returned to the venous circulation. In addition, the lymphatic system plays a key role in dietary lipid absorption and trafficking leucocytes and peripheral antigens.

Lymphatic malformations (LMs) are congenital abnormalities of lymphatic vessels. Although the exact incidence of LMs has not been well established, the estimated prevalence is approximately 1 in 4,000 (1). They can be solitary or multifocal. Most are common cystic LMs. As well as causing disruption of the lymphatic system, LMs can cause local disruption of adjacent tissues and organs. Rarer, complex lymphatic anomalies may also infiltrate other critical structures, leading to significant morbidity. Solitary LMs are discussed in Chapter 8.

Complex lymphatic anomalies (CLA) are either multifocal or involve central conducting lymphatic channels. The progressive and infiltrative nature of these lymphatic lesions make treatment extremely challenging and leads to significant morbidity and mortality in affected patients. Previously termed 'lymphangiomatosis', the classification of CLAs has been refined in recent years into four subtypes:

- Generalised lymphatic anomaly (GLA)
- Kaposiform lymphatic anomaly (KLA)
- Gorham–Stout disease (GSD)
- Central conducting lymphatic anomaly (CCLA)

Clinical presentation varies widely between individuals, depending on the anatomical location and extent of lymphatic involvement. There is often significant overlap between these subtypes, often making diagnosis challenging.

## CLASSIFICATION OF COMPLEX LYMPHATIC ANOMALIES

GLA describes multifocal, proliferative lymphatic lesions that can affect the soft tissues and any organ system, including bone. Common organs involved include liver, spleen, lungs, bone, and soft tissues. KLA is really a subtype of GLA which has been defined histologically by the presence of Kaposiform spindle-shaped lymphatic endothelial cells. Differentiation between GLA and KLA can be challenging. Of note, a single biopsy may not demonstrate pathognomonic spindle-shaped lymphatic endothelial cells. Other differentiating features suggested to favour a diagnosis of KLA include mediastinal involvement, a refractory coagulopathy often with profound thrombocytopenia and hypofibrinogenaemia, characteristic imaging features, and an aggressive clinical picture, often with a poor prognosis. The mechanism by which the coagulopathy occurs is not clear.

DOI: 10.1201/9781003257417-9

GSD, previously termed disappearing or vanishing bone disease, is distinguished by progressive bone destruction and resorption. Although GLA, KLA, and CCLA may also have pathological bone involvement, bone involvement in GSD is characterised by peri-osseous expansion of lymphatic channels, resulting in progressive loss of cortical bone. The majority of patients will also have peri-osseous infiltration of soft tissue. GSD may involve adjacent bones, although involvement is not always continuous and may skip joints and soft tissues. GSD can occur anywhere but frequently involves the axial skeleton. When involving the thorax, GSD may be complicated by pleural effusions or by cerebrospinal fluid leak when affecting the base of the skull.

CCLA, or channel-type, previously termed lymphangiectasia, is characterised by grossly dilated or obstructed lymphatic channels and typically results in impaired lymph clearance or leakage of lymph into body cavities. This can manifest as pleural and/or pericardial effusions, ascites, or peripheral lymphoedema. When the gut is involved, as in intestinal lymphangiectasia, this results in a protein-losing enteropathy with hypoalbuminaemia and hypogammaglobulinaemia. These characteristics are frequently observed in CCLA but can also be a feature of any CLA.

# GENETIC BASIS OF COMPLEX LYMPHATIC ANOMALY

Advances in genetic sequencing technology and ease of access to next-generation sequencing, over recent years, have accelerated the identification of causative pathogenic genetic variants in CLA. Many of the genetic variants identified are somatic in nature, as commonly observed across the majority of vascular anomalies. However, recently, germline variants have been described in severe phenotypes of CCLA, which present antenatally and are often fatal. Identified genetic causes are summarised in Table 9.1.

**TABLE 9.1** Genetic basis and inheritance of CLA

| CLA Subtype | Gene Implicated/Mode of Inheritance |
|---|---|
| Generalised lymphatic anomaly (GLA) | Somatic activating mutations in *PIK3CA* (2) |
| Kaposiform lymphatic anomaly (KLA) | Somatic activating mutations in *NRAS* (3, 4) and *CBL* (5) |
| Gorham–Stout disease (GSD) | Somatic activating mutations in *KRAS* (6) |
| Central conducting LA (CCLA) | Somatic activating mutations in *ARAF* (7)<br>Germline heterozygous mutation in *EPHB4* (8)<br>Germline recessive bi-allelic mutations in *MDFIC* (9) |

# CLINICAL PRESENTATION

The multifocal nature of CLA leads to a broad phenotypic spectrum with clinical presentation dictated by anatomical location and extent of disease. Age at clinical presentation varies widely, with some cases diagnosed antenatally, for example, by detection of visceral or soft-tissue lesions compatible with this diagnosis or pleural, pericardial, or ascitic effusions. Many patients present later in life, including in adulthood, with acute or chronic pulmonary insufficiency.

Overlapping clinical features across the four subtypes are common and can lead to diagnostic confusion. Helpful differentiating clinical features of each subtype are highlighted in Table 9.2.

Organ-specific clinical features found in all types of CLA are outlined in Table 9.3.

# CLINICAL ASSESSMENT AND INITIAL INVESTIGATIONS

## CLINICAL EXAMINATION

Owing to the multifocal and often inconspicuous nature of CLA, any child suspected to have this diagnosis should undergo a full system physical examination. This should include documentation of growth parameters and basic clinical measurements such as heart rate, respiratory rate, oxygen saturations, and blood pressure. A full cutaneous examination should reference the presence or absence of any soft-tissue mass, generalised or localised lymphoedema, bruising or purpuric lesions, and any suspected superficial vascular lesions of the skin, often presenting as purple/red/brown/pink confluent lesions with or without lymphatic blebs or superficial verrucous lesions (Figure 9.1). Areas of hyperpigmentation may also

**TABLE 9.2** Differentiating clinical features of each CLA subtype

| Differentiating clinical features of CLA subtypes |
| --- |

**Generalised lymphatic anomaly (GLA)**
- Diffuse or multicentric invasive lesions in multiple organs, including the bones, liver, spleen, lungs, and soft tissues.
- Bony lesions typically lytic and not involving the cortex.

**Kaposiform lymphatic anomaly (KLA)**
Subtype of GLA; main differentiating features:
- Histological presence of foci of Kaposiform spindle-shaped lymphatic endothelial cells (although not seen universally across lymphatic lesions, so they may not be evident).
- Thrombocytopenia.
- MRI signal differs from GLA.
- More likely to involve the mediastinum.
- Aggressive course, poor prognosis.

**Gorham–Stout disease (GSD)**
- Peri-osseous expansion of lymphatic channels resulting in progressive loss of cortical bone, with or without peri-osseous infiltration of soft tissue.
- Regional disease, i.e., localised to adjacent bones, although may skip joints and soft tissues.
- Frequently involving the axial skeleton with a predilection for long, flat bones.

**Central conducting lymphatic anomaly (CCLA)**
- Dilated central conducting lymphatic vessels.
- Presentation can include:
  - Protein-losing enteropathy.
  - Pleural/pericardial effusions.
  - Ascites.
  - Peripheral oedema.
  - Fetal hydrops.

be observed. Any area of asymmetric growth or limb length/girth discrepancy should be documented. Musculoskeletal examination should include examination to identify any visible skeletal deformity, including scoliosis, and note of the range of motion of involved joints. Abdominal examination should be performed to look for any organomegaly or ascites. Cardiorespiratory examination should focus on assessment for any clinical evidence of pleural or pericardial effusions.

Clinical photography should be taken at baseline and may be useful to monitor cutaneous lymphatic lesions and obvious skeletal deformity.

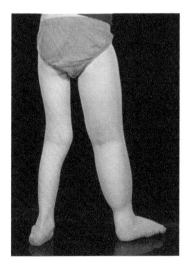

FIGURE 9.1 A 5-year-old male with a multifocal lymphatic anomaly involving the abdomen, pelvis, retroperitoneum, spleen, spine, paraspinal soft tissue, and the right leg.

**TABLE 9.3** Organ-specific presenting features of CLA and proposed investigations

| System | Clinical Presentation | Useful Investigations | Subtypes |
|---|---|---|---|
| Skin/soft tissue | Palpable soft tissue mass<br>Lymphangioma circumscriptum<br>Lymphoedema<br>Hyperpigmentation | Ultrasound/MRI<br>Lymphangiography<br>Skin biopsy for histological markers of lymphatic malformations (e.g., PROX1, D2-40, LYVE1) | Can be present or absent across all subtypes, but most frequently observed in GLA and KLA |
| Haematological | Localised or disseminated intravascular coagulopathy | Full blood count and clotting screen<br>Fibrinogen level<br>D-dimer level | Coagulopathy most severe in KLA |
| Gastrointestinal | Protein-losing enteropathy secondary to intestinal lymphangiectasia | Serum albumin level<br>Immunoglobulin levels | |
| Bone | Pathological fracture<br>Pain<br>Deformity<br>Scoliosis | Plain radiographs<br>MRI<br>Metabolic bone profile | Lytic lesions in GLA and KLA<br>Progressive resorption of cortical bone in GSD<br>Contiguous involvement across joints in GSD |
| Respiratory | Pleural effusions<br>Restrictive lung disease<br>Respiratory insufficiency | Plain radiographs<br>MRI<br>Lymphangiography<br>Pulmonary function tests | Any, but a key feature of KLA and CCLA |
| Cardiovascular | Pericardial effusions<br>Cardiac tamponade<br>Cardiac arrest | Echocardiogram<br>MRI | Any, but a key feature of KLA and CCLA |

## LABORATORY TESTS

A full blood count should be carried out at baseline to look for thrombocytopenia, anaemia, or lymphopenia, and coagulation studies to look for evidence of disseminated intravascular coagulation. D-dimer levels may be elevated, and trends in D-dimer levels may be used to monitor progress, as single values are often not helpful in isolation. Recent studies have proposed angiopoietin 2 levels as a clinical biomarker of disease activity in KLA (10). This can be measured from serum in specialised laboratories with age/sex-based reference ranges recently described. Haematological considerations for CLA are discussed in more detail in Chapter 3.

In cases of visceral, gut, or bone involvement, serial liver function tests are recommended, including serum albumin, immunoglobulins, renal function, and a bone profile. For children with lymphopaenia, we would recommend measurement of lymphocyte subsets and referral to a paediatric immunology service.

## BIOPSY

Biopsy of affected tissue should be performed, when possible, to confirm the histological diagnosis and to enable genetic studies which may help to characterise subtype and guide medical therapy. If there is cutaneous involvement, this can be performed via a simple skin punch biopsy, although even this may be complicated by an underlying coagulopathy or by subsequent lymph leak and infection. Deep lesions should be biopsied by a surgeon or interventional radiologist.

# IMAGING

Patients in whom CLA is suspected should undergo multimodality imaging tailored to the clinical presentation and suspected areas of disease involvement. Whole-body magnetic resonance imaging (MRI) is useful as the first screening imaging for suspected CLA. It is a highly sensitive technique to identify effusions (pleural, pericardial, or ascites), soft tissue mass, and bone lesions but will not provide detailed imaging of each region. On MRI, KLA has similar features to GLA but also can include enhancing, infiltrative soft tissue masses in the mediastinum and retroperitoneum (11, 12) (Figures 9.2–9.4).

The bone lesions in GSD are usually focal or contiguous. GLA may involve separate, distinct areas and significantly affect the strength and quality of the bone before any symptoms arise (12). For bony disease, plain radiographs are useful for disease monitoring. Assessment of the lung parenchymal changes, which can occur with CCLA and KLA, should be made initially on chest radiography and computed tomography (CT). Ultrasound should be used to assess any soft tissue lesions and effusions. Soft tissue lesions may demonstrate enlarged hypoechoic compressible channels with absent blood flow on colour Doppler.

Functional imaging is also useful in the diagnosis of CLA. This takes the form of

- Pedal lymphoscintigraphy using Tc 99 m sulphur colloid with and without single-photon emission computed tomography (SPECT), which is useful for the peripheral lymphatic system both for lower and upper extremities, and/or
- Intranodal dynamic magnetic resonance lymphangiography (MRL), which evaluates the central conducting lymphatics (from the pelvic lymphatics to the site of drainage of the thoracic duct) (12)

MRL involves heavily T2-weighted MRI sequences to demonstrate fluid-filled lymphatic channels and provide anatomical detail, followed by direct intranodal injection of gadolinium contrast medium both immediately prior to and during sequence acquisition to delineate lymphatic flow. This technique has been used with increased frequency instead of conventional lymphangiography in the past decade.

# MEDICAL MANAGEMENT

A number of medical therapies have been reported to show efficacy in CLA in single case reports or small cases series.

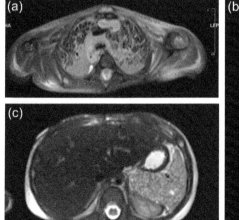
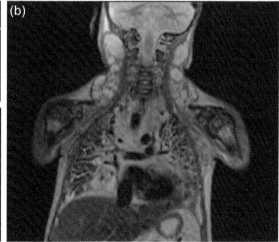

FIGURE 9.2 A 14-month-old child who presented with a large pericardial effusion and was eventually diagnosed with KLA. T2-weighted axial (a) and coronal (b) MRI images of the chest demonstrate soft tissue thickening of the superior mediastinum with interlobular septal thickening in the lungs. The coronal image also shows lesions in the humeral metaphysis. T2-weighted axial image of the upper abdomen (c) showing innumerable cystic lesions in the spleen.

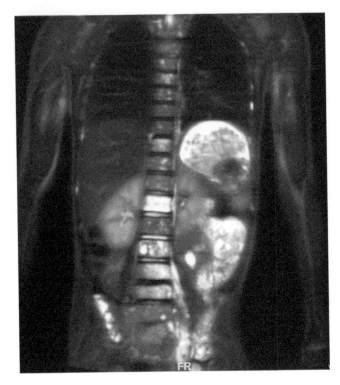

FIGURE 9.3 A 5-year-old child with GLA. MRI T2-weighted coronal image demonstrates multilevel vertebral disease and disease in both ilium bones.

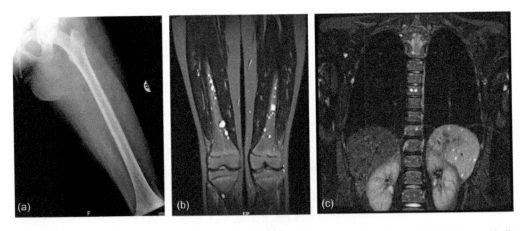

FIGURE 9.4 A 13-year-old child with GLA. AP radiograph of the left femur (a) shows well-defined lytic lesions in the femur. MRI T2-weighted coronal image through the thighs, (b) also demonstrates high signal well-defined extremity lesions and (c), through the chest and upper abdomen, shows lesions in the vertebrae and spleen.

Sirolimus, an mTOR inhibitor, thus, acting downstream of p110alpha, was used successfully in the treatment of LMs for several years prior to knowledge of its underlying genetic basis. A Phase II trial demonstrated the safety and efficacy of sirolimus for patients with complex vascular anomalies, including a partial response in 7/7 patients with GLA, 1/3 patients with GSD, and 6/7 patients with KLA (13), with a further study from the same group demonstrating a response in at least one aspect of disease in 15/18 patients with either GLA or GSD (14). Recently, alpelisib, a specific inhibitor of p110alpha and, therefore, a more directly targeted therapy for somatic mutations in *PIK3CA*, was demonstrated to be safe and effective in a compassionate-use series of 19 adults with *PIK3CA*-related overgrowth syndrome, including those with significant lymphatic components to their disease (15). Small case series have since demonstrated efficacy of alpelisib in solitary large LMs, including some cases refractory to sirolimus. (16, 17). The role of alpelisib, specifically in *PIK3CA*-related GLA, has yet to be established.

There is good evidence from numerous case series that the use of bisphosphonates can reduce pain in CLA with bone involvement, particularly in combination with sirolimus. Paediatric endocrine support should be sought for bisphosphonate treatment. There is an emerging body of evidence suggesting the MEK inhibitor trametinib is a promising targeted treatment for MAPK pathway-related CLA, with a number of positive reports of resolution or reduction of disease in *ARAF* (18), *CBL* (5), and *NRAS* (19) CLA. A number of these cases exhibited severe, extensive phenotypes with significant respiratory insufficiency refractory to treatment with sirolimus, with dramatic remodelling of the lymphatic vasculature confirmed by lymphangiogram following commencement of MEKi. This is highly encouraging, although these are single case reports, and long-term data on safety and efficacy from a larger cohort is not available.

These recent advances emphasise the importance of routine tissue genotyping in all patients with CLA to enable personalised targeted treatments when possible.

# RADIOLOGICAL AND SURGICAL MANAGEMENT

Medical management is the mainstay of CLA treatment. Interventional treatments of CLA are aimed at relief of symptoms and local control. Symptomatic pleural effusions or ascites can be symptomatically managed by serial drainage. For pleural effusions, pleurodesis may provide some benefit. Ascites can be shunted to the venous circulation; however, this is often complicated by mechanical shunt blockages. At specific sites of lymphatic leakage, targeted embolisation of lymphatic channels with ethiodised oil (Lipiodol®) can be performed; however, recurrence usually occurs. There is a limited role for sclerotherapy, for example, in managing focal cutaneous lymphatic fluid leaks (20). When lymphangiography demonstrates thoracic duct dysfunction and failure of lymphatic fluid to empty into the venous circulation, surgical lymphatico-venous anastomosis can be attempted (21).

---

## KEY MESSAGES

* CLAs are either multifocal or involve central conducting lymphatic channels; clinical presentation varies widely, and diagnosis can be challenging.

* CLA is classified into four subtypes: GLA, KLA, GSD, and CCLA; there is, however, significant phenotypic overlap between types.

* CLAs are predominantly caused by somatic activating variants of the RAS-MAPK pathway; however, germline recessive variants have been described.

* Any child suspected to have a CLA should undergo a full system physical examination, blood tests, and a biopsy when possible.

* Whole-body MRI is useful as the first screening imaging for suspected CLA; the lung parenchymal changes which can occur with CCLA and KLA should be imaged with plain chest radiography and CT.

* Functional imaging is also useful in the diagnosis of CLA; pedal lymphoscintigraphy is used to image disease in the extremities, while intranodal dynamic magnetic

resonance lymphangiography (MRL) evaluates the central conducting lymphatics (from the pelvis to the thoracic duct).

- Due to the multifocal and infiltrative nature of CLAs, medical management is the mainstay of treatment.

- Interventional treatment of CLAs, such as pleural drains and pleurodesis, are aimed at relief of symptoms and local control.

- Targeted embolisation of lymphatic leaks, sclerotherapy, and surgical lymphaticovenous anastomoses can be attempted in selected cases, but outcomes are highly variable.

# REFERENCES

1. Gallagher, J.R., Martini, J., Carroll, S., Small, A., and Teng, J. (2022). Annual prevalence estimation of lymphatic malformation with a cutaneous component: Observational study of a national representative sample of physicians. *Orphanet J Rare Dis* 17, 192.
2. Rodriguez-Laguna, L., Agra, N., Ibañez, K., Oliva-Molina, G., Gordo, G., Khurana, N., Hominick, D., Beato, M., Colmenero, I., Herranz, G., et al. (2019). Somatic activating mutations in PIK3CA cause generalized lymphatic anomaly. *J Exp Med* 216, 407–418.
3. Barclay, S.F., Inman, K.W., Luks, V.L., McIntyre, J.B., Al-Ibraheemi, A., Church, A.J., Perez-Atayde, A.R., Mangray, S., Jeng, M., Kreimer, S.R., et al. (2019). A somatic activating NRAS variant associated with kaposiform lymphangiomatosis. *Genet Med: Off J Am J Med Genet* 21, 1517–1524.
4. Manevitz-Mendelson, E., Leichner, G.S., Barel, O., Davidi-Avrahami, I., Ziv-Strasser, L., Eyal, E., Pessach, I., Rimon, U., Barzilai, A., Hirshberg, A., et al. (2018). Somatic NRAS mutation in patient with generalized lymphatic anomaly. *Angiogenesis* 21, 287–298.
5. Foster, J.B., Li, D., March, M.E., Sheppard, S.E., Adams, D.M., Hakonarson, H., and Dori, Y. (2020). Kaposiform lymphangiomatosis effectively treated with MEK inhibition. *EMBO Mol Med* 12, e12324.
6. Nozawa, A., Ozeki, M., Niihori, T., Suzui, N., Miyazaki, T., and Aoki, Y. (2020). A somatic activating KRAS variant identified in an affected lesion of a patient with Gorham-Stout disease. *J Hum Genet* 65, 995–1001.
7. Li, D., March, M.E., Gutierrez-Uzquiza, A., Kao, C., Seiler, C., Pinto, E., Matsuoka, L.S., Battig, M.R., Bhoj, E.J., Wenger, T.L., et al. (2019). ARAF recurrent mutation causes central conducting lymphatic anomaly treatable with a MEK inhibitor. *Nat Med* 25, 1116–1122.
8. Li, D., Wenger, T.L., Seiler, C., March, M.E., Gutierrez-Uzquiza, A., Kao, C., Bhoj, E., Tian, L., Rosenbach, M., Liu, Y., et al. (2018). Pathogenic variant in EPHB4 results in central conducting lymphatic anomaly. *Hum Mol Genet* 27, 3233–3245.
9. Byrne, A.B., Brouillard, P., Sutton, D.L., Kazenwadel, J., Montazaribarforoushi, S., Secker, G.A., Oszmiana, A., Babic, M., Betterman, K.L., Brautigan, P.J., et al. (2022). Pathogenic variants in MDFIC cause recessive central conducting lymphatic anomaly with lymphedema. *Sci Transl Med* 14, eabm4869.
10. Le Cras, T.D., Mobberley-Schuman, P.S., Broering, M., Fei, L., Trenor, C.C., 3rd, and Adams, D.M. (2017). Angiopoietins as serum biomarkers for lymphatic anomalies. *Angiogenesis* 20, 163–173.
11. Goyal, P., Alomari, A.I., Kozakewich, H.P., Trenor, C.C., 3rd, Perez-Atayde, A.R., Fishman, S.J., Greene, A.K., Shaikh, R., and Chaudry, G. (2016). Imaging features of kaposiform lymphangiomatosis. *Pediatr Radiol* 46, 1282–1290.
12. Iacobas, I., Adams, D.M., Pimpalwar, S., Phung, T., Blei, F., Burrows, P., Lopez-Gutierrez, J.C., Levine, M.A., and Trenor, C.C., 3rd. (2020). Multidisciplinary guidelines for initial evaluation of complicated lymphatic anomalies-expert opinion consensus. *Pediatr Blood Cancer* 67, e28036.
13. Adams, D.M., Trenor, C.C., 3rd, Hammill, A.M., Vinks, A.A., Patel, M.N., Chaudry, G., Wentzel, M.S., Mobberley-Schuman, P.S., Campbell, L.M., Brookbank, C., et al. (2016). Efficacy and safety of sirolimus in the treatment of complicated vascular anomalies. *Pediatrics* 137, e20153257.
14. Ricci, K.W., Hammill, A.M., Mobberley-Schuman, P., Nelson, S.C., Blatt, J., Bender, J.L.G., McCuaig, C.C., Synakiewicz, A., Frieden, I.J., and Adams, D.M. (2019). Efficacy of systemic sirolimus in the treatment of generalized lymphatic anomaly and Gorham-Stout disease. *Pediatr Blood Cancer* 66, e27614.
15. Venot, Q., Blanc, T., Rabia, S.H., Berteloot, L., Ladraa, S., Duong, J.P., Blanc, E., Johnson, S.C., Hoguin, C., Boccara, O., et al. (2018). Targeted therapy in patients with PIK3CA-related overgrowth syndrome. *Nature* 558, 540–546.
16. Delestre, F., Venot, Q., Bayard, C., Fraissenon, A., Ladraa, S., Hoguin, C., Chapelle, C., Yamaguchi, J., Cassaca, R., Zerbib, L., et al. (2021). Alpelisib administration reduced lymphatic malformations in a mouse model and in patients. *Sci Transl Med* 13, eabg0809.
17. Wenger, T.L., Ganti, S., Bull, C., Lutsky, E., Bennett, J.T., Zenner, K., Jensen, D.M., Dmyterko, V., Mercan, E., Shivaram, G.M., et al. (2022). Alpelisib for the treatment of PIK3CA-related head and neck lymphatic malformations and overgrowth. *Genet Med: Off J Am J Med Genet* 24, 2318–2328.
18. Li, D., March, M.E., Gutierrez-Uzquiza, A., Kao, C., Seiler, C., Pinto, E., Matsuoka, L.S., Battig, M.R., Bhoj, E.J., Wenger, T.L., et al. (2019). ARAF recurrent mutation causes central conducting lymphatic anomaly treatable with a MEK inhibitor. *Nat Med* 25, 1116–1122.
19. Chowers, G., Abebe-Campino, G., Golan, H., Vivante, A., Greenberger, S., Soudack, M., Barkai, G., Fox-Fisher, I., Li, D., March, M., et al. (2022). Treatment of severe kaposiform lymphangiomatosis positive for NRAS mutation by MEK inhibition. *Pediatr Res*. doi: 10.1038/s41390-022-01986-0.

20. Snyder, E.J., Sarma, A., Borst, A.J., and Tekes, A. (2022). Lymphatic anomalies in children: Update on imaging diagnosis, genetics, and treatment. *AJR Am J Roentgenol* 218, 1089–1101.
21. Taghinia, A.H., Upton, J., Trenor, C.C., 3rd, Alomari, A.I., Lillis, A.P., Shaikh, R., Burrows, P.E., and Fishman, S.J. (2019). Lymphaticovenous bypass of the thoracic duct for the treatment of chylous leak in central conducting lymphatic anomalies. *J Pediatr Surg* 54, 562–568.

# Venous Malformations

**10**

Kishore Minhas and Maanasa Polubothu

## PATHOGENESIS AND GENETIC BASIS

Venous malformations (VMs) occur due to mutations in the genes which code for the growth and development of veins and lead to venous dysplasia. This dysplasia causes the affected veins to have an abnormal morphology, to be abnormally located, or to be abnormally numerous. These genetic mutations are almost always somatic, and only rarely do VMs arise as a result of an inherited genetic mutation, in which case, there may be a family history of vascular malformations (1, 2).

More than 50% of sporadic VMs are caused by somatic mutations in the gene *TEK,* the gene encoding the endothelial cell tyrosine kinase receptor TIE-2, which is thought to result in ligand independent phosphorylation of the receptor and activation of the downstream PI3K-AKT-mTOR pathway (3). Of the remaining sporadic VMs, approximately half are caused by somatic activating mutations in *PIK3CA*, the gene encoding the catalytic p110α subunit of PI3K (4). As discussed in other chapters, somatic activating mutations in *PIK3CA* give rise to many simple or mixed vascular anomalies and overgrowth syndromes by activation of the PI3K-AKT pathway, a key growth pathway.

VMs are congenital, being present at birth, although, in some cases, not clinically detectable, and grow in line with the growth of the patient. They are sensitive to hormonal changes, demonstrating more rapid growth during puberty and pregnancy (5). The exact reason for rapid growth during puberty and pregnancy is not completely understood.

## CLINICAL PRESENTATION

VMs are often mistaken for other vascular anomalies, particularly infantile haemangiomas. However, unlike infantile haemangiomas, VMs are congenital and present from birth and do not demonstrate the natural history of rapid growth during the first few months of life before undergoing involution, nor do they have a solid tumoral component (6). However, if small, VMs may not be clinically appreciable and may only be discovered later in life when they increase in size or become painful.

VMs can occur anywhere in the body but are relatively more common in the head and neck region and in the limbs and can occur in any tissue or anatomical space (1). They can be localised but can also be diffuse and trans-spatial, crossing multiple anatomical territories. Congenital overgrowth syndromes are characterised by excessive proliferation of a region of the body, and a subset of these overgrowth syndromes is associated with vascular anomalies including VMs. Overgrowth syndromes are discussed in detail in Chapter 12.

Patients with VMs can present with a variety of clinical symptoms, including pain and swelling, thrombophlebitis, coagulopathy, and aesthetic disfigurement. Large VMs, which may affect an entire limb, or which may have an extensive intra-articular component, may cause functional problems. Pain or discomfort is the most frequent presenting complaint. Patients typically describe pain and swelling at the site of the malformation that worsens toward the end of the day, after vigorous exercise, during an intercurrent illness, or in warm weather. Pain or stiffness is also commonly reported on waking, presumably due to prolonged stasis of blood within the malformation while the patient has been sleeping.

104

DOI: 10.1201/9781003257417-10

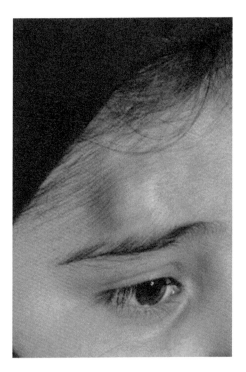

FIGURE 10.1 Typical clinical appearance of a venous malformation.

On clinical examination, the VM is typically soft and compressible, and there may be a bluish discolouration of the overlying skin, depending on how superficial the malformation is (7) (Figure 10.1). If intralesional phleboliths or thrombus are present, the malformation may feel firm and non-compressible. If the lesion is quiescent, it is typically non-tender on palpation. However, if acutely inflamed or infected, the presence of thrombophlebitis may make the lesion painful to touch.

The veins within a VM are morphologically abnormal, and blood flow through those veins is, typically, very slow and, in some cases, there is no flow at all, manifesting as venous stasis. Subsequently, this can lead to the formation of thrombus within the VM. Intralesional thrombus is usually confined to the malformation and can be painful. Large VMs may lead to the development of such a large volume of thrombus that it may give rise to a consumptive coagulopathy and lead to abnormal clotting elsewhere in the body (see Chapter 3).

Large VMs can also cause problems because of their size. As there is slow flow or stasis of blood within the abnormal veins, it can cause the malformation to swell, particularly in regions of the body where the flow of venous blood is against gravity, such as the lower limbs. This can cause pain and discomfort, particularly after long periods of standing or walking. This swelling or discomfort is usually alleviated by rest, elevating the affected area, or using a compression garment to 'squeeze' blood out of these dysplastic venous lakes.

Typically, patients or their caregivers will describe the VM becoming visibly more noticeable on exertion. An example of this is when a young child cries or when a child undertakes strenuous physical activity, such as sports. This visible accentuation occurs due to increased blood flow to the malformation and filling of the venous channels during increased physical exertion.

VMs that are close to, or extend into, a joint can bleed into the joint space. Repeated bleeding of the malformation into the intra-articular space can cause premature arthritis and the development of debilitating joint problems in later life.

VMs usually grow in proportion with the child's growth, but there can be periods of acute swelling, such as after an episode of trauma or periods of accelerated growth which occur due to hormonal influences, such as during puberty or pregnancy.

## DIAGNOSIS AND IMAGING

VMs can be suspected based on the clinical history and physical examination but usually require imaging to confirm the diagnosis and rule out more sinister pathologies.

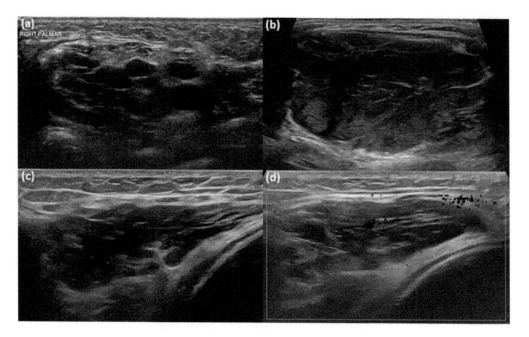

FIGURE 10.2 (a) Ultrasound image of a venous malformation of the palm of the hand, demonstrating poorly defined serpiginous, anechoic venous spaces within the soft tissues; (b) ultrasound image of a well-defined venous malformation of the lower limb, demonstrating low level echoes within the venous spaces, suggesting the presence of echogenic material, often seen with stasis of blood (i.e., very slow flow); (c and d) ultrasound images of a venous malformation demonstrate absence of significant flow on Doppler assessment (d), indicative of a slow-flow venous malformation.

Ultrasound is the first-line imaging test. Ultrasound is readily available, does not confer ionising radiation, and can be performed in the setting of an outpatient clinic review. On sonographic assessment, VMs typically appear as dysplastic, compressible, venous channels without an associated solid soft tissue mass. Typically, the venous blood flow through these dysplastic veins is so slow that colour signal may not be evident on Doppler interrogation (Figure 10.2). In fact, the presence of plentiful colour signal should make one question the diagnosis of a VM. A phlebolith (calcified clot), seen as a well-defined echogenic entity that casts an acoustic shadow, may be seen within the malformation on ultrasound and is a defining feature (Figure 10.3).

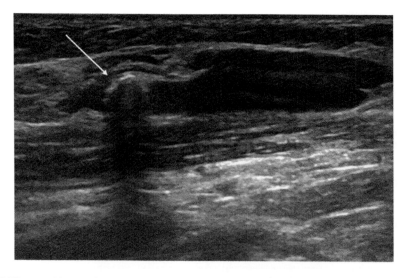

FIGURE 10.3 Ultrasound image shows a hypoechoic venous space containing a well circumscribed echogenic entity (white arrow) that casts an acoustic shadow. This is typical of an intralesional phlebolith.

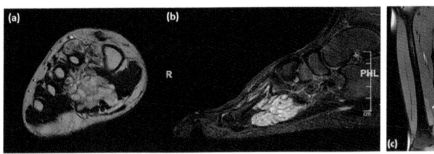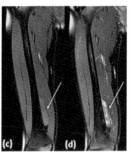

FIGURE 10.4 (a) T2-weighted axial MRI image shows a trans-spatial, hyperintense lesion involving the muscles of the plantar aspect of the foot; (b) T2-weighted fat-supressed sagittal MRI image shows that the same lesion remains hyperintense (bright) relative to the surrounding soft tissue structures, differentiating it from fat and increasing the conspicuity of the lesion; (c and d) T1 fat saturated pre- and post-contrast enhanced MRI images in the coronal plane show a venous malformation of the medial aspect (white arrow) of the distal thigh that is isointense relative to muscle and demonstrates heterogenous enhancement on the enhanced image. This is typical of a venous malformation, but enhancement can vary depending on the timing of contrast administration.

Magnetic resonance imaging (MRI) is a useful adjunct to a focused ultrasound examination (Figure 10.4). It can further delineate the extent of extensive VMs; can be used for regions which are difficult to see on ultrasound, such as within the joint space; be used to monitor response to treatment; and be used when the diagnosis is not certain on ultrasound alone. On MRI, VMs appear hyperintense on water sensitive sequences (T2, STIR), and phleboliths will appear as areas of signal dropout (8). Post-contrast sequences can be difficult to interpret, depending on the imaging delay following the administration of intravenous contrast. On immediate post-contrast sequences, there may be no or only limited and heterogeneous contrast enhancement, as the blood flow is so slow that the venous spaces have not filled with contrast. Delayed post-contrast sequences will demonstrate more homogenous enhancement, as more time has passed for contrast to fill the venous spaces. The additional benefit of cross-sectional imaging is that it allows for assessment of the deep venous system in the evaluation of limb VMs. For example, if a deep venous system is not present in a lower limb, then treatment of a VM which comprises the superficial venous system may be contraindicated so as to avoid venous hypertension and post-thrombotic syndrome.

CT is rarely required in the evaluation of a VM, as it is inferior to MRI in terms of imaging resolution and confers unnecessary ionising radiation.

Similarly, plain radiographs are seldom required but can be useful in assessing the degree of joint damage in cases of VMs which have intra-articular involvement (Figure 10.5) and can be used to detect calcified phleboliths.

On occasion, a VM may have atypical ultrasound and MRI features. In these cases, it may be necessary to undertake a biopsy to exclude more sinister pathology before embarking on treatment. Our institutional preference is to undertake a percutaneous, image-guided, needle biopsy, as it is minimally invasive and yields a sufficient volume of tissue to make a diagnosis.

## HISTOPATHOLOGY

Histologically, VMs are predominantly composed of irregular and dysplastic venous-type channels, lined by flat endothelium and surrounded by an abnormal layer of smooth muscle that is often focally absent or irregular. Venous vessels vary in number, size, and distribution but often exhibit secondary changes, such as thrombi and organisation, which may form mineralised phleboliths over time. The vascular endothelial cells in VM are highlighted by CD31/34 but show no other specific features. Smooth muscle actin highlights the pericytes and smooth muscle within the wall. The Ki-67 proliferative index is low and lymphatic endothelial markers are negative (Figure 10.6).

## TREATMENT

The management of VMs requires a multidisciplinary team approach and can involve input from a number of paediatric specialties including, but not limited to, paediatric dermatology, haematology, interventional radiology, and plastic surgery as well as allied health professionals such as physiotherapists and occupational therapists. The options for treatment depend on the size and location of the malformation and the symptoms that it causes.

Treatment

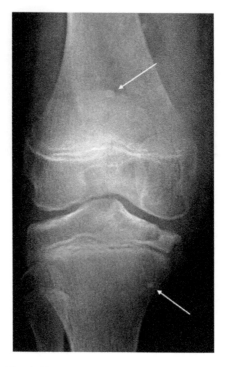

FIGURE 10.5 Plain radiograph of the right knee in a patient with an intra-articular venous malformation shows radiographic features of joint destruction including non-uniform joint space narrowing and subchondral cyst formation. Tiny calcific densities are also present (white arrows) in keeping with phleboliths.

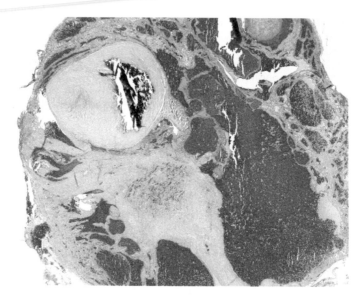

FIGURE 10.6 Photomicrograph of venous malformation with organising haemorrhage and phlebolith. Original magnification x12.5 H&E.

## CONSERVATIVE

For VMs that are entirely asymptomatic, the only management that may be required is reassuring the patient and their family of the diagnosis and its benign nature, as, in many cases, the malformation may initially have been detected as a lump and raised concern of a more sinister pathology such as malignancy.

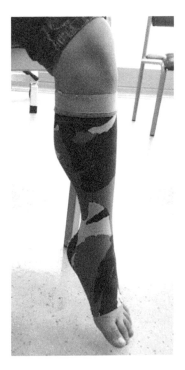

FIGURE 10.7 A custom-made compression garment for a patient with a left calf venous malformation.

VMs which are only mildly symptomatic, such as those which are only intermittently painful and not disrupting activities of daily living, may be able to be managed with conservative measures alone, at least in the first instance. Conservative measures primarily include lifestyle changes, the use of compression garments for extremity VMs, and analgesic medicines when required.

Lifestyle adjustments should be tailored to the individual patient, such as the avoidance of contact sports. However, one could consider the inability to partake in normal activities of life, such as regular absence from school or the inability to take part in school sports, as an indication for more active intervention.

A graded compression garment acts to 'squeeze' blood out of the malformation and, in doing so, prevents the pooling of blood within the malformation which can help reduce pain and swelling and minimise the likelihood of static venous blood giving rise to intralesional thrombus formation. Although variably tolerated, patients should be encouraged to wear their compression garments for as much of the day as practically possible. The compression garment should be updated regularly to account for the child's growth, as an overly tight-fitting garment can, itself, be uncomfortable and a loosely fitted garment can be ineffective (Figure 10.7).

Infrequent bouts of pain can be managed with simple analgesia such as paracetamol and non-steroidal anti-inflammatory medicines and the use of heat or ice packs. More frequent bouts of pain and the use of regular and increasing amounts of analgesia should be considered an indication for more invasive treatments.

If there is evidence of localised intravascular coagulation within a VM, an entity which reflects the localised consumption of clotting factors causing a rise in D-dimers and a fall in serum fibrinogen, anticoagulation medicines may be prescribed. This should be done under the auspices of a haematologist and will require regular blood tests to monitor the coagulopathy (9) (see Chapter 3).

## SCLEROTHERAPY

The indication for interventional treatment for VMs includes, but is not limited to, regular episodes of pain requiring the use of regular analgesia and disturbance of daily activities, such as prolonged time off school or the inability to partake in sports or recreational activities.

Percutaneous, image-guided sclerotherapy is generally regarded as the first-line treatment for the management of VMs. Its purpose is not to cure the VM but, rather, to shrink and/or limit the growth of the malformation so that it is less painful, less troublesome to joints, and less unsightly. Sclerotherapy involves the image-guided injection of a medicine, or combination of medicines, into the abnormal veins of the malformation which irritates them and encourages them to become inflamed and, in turn, to scar down and shrink. It may take several sequential sclerotherapy treatments of a VM before improvements are evident.

There are numerous medicines which have been used as sclerosants. Historically, absolute ethanol and OK-432 (Picibanil™) were commonly used. However, ethanol is now infrequently used because of its relatively high complication rates, the risk of severe pain, and the weight-based volume limitation in children (10). OK-432 is now less readily available.

The more commonly used sclerosants in current practice are sodium tetradecyl sulfate (STS) (5, 11) and bleomycin. STS is an anionic detergent-based sclerosant. It is available in several concentrations up to a 3%. Bleomycin is a cytostatic antibiotic derivative and primarily utilised as a chemotherapeutic drug. Its exact mechanism for action as a sclerosant is not completely understood, but there is the suggestion that it works by disrupting endothelial cross-linkage junction cells as well as inducing endothelial mesenchymal transition, leading to fibroblast-like transformation (12).

Most sclerotherapy procedures in children are performed under general anaesthetic, although mature adolescent patients may tolerate technically straightforward procedures with the use of conscious sedation and local anaesthetic only. A preliminary ultrasound is performed to map out the malformation and plan the treatment. Considerations at this stage will include the number of needles required to access the malformation and the length of those needles to access the deepest components of the malformation. Using a sterile technique, the venous spaces are then accessed under ultrasound guidance using the appropriate number of needles to obtain coverage of all parts of the malformation (Figure 10.8). In very large VMs, the operator may wish to focus each treatment on one part of the malformation and concentrate future treatments on other parts of the VM. The choice of needle is at the discretion of the operator but, typically, includes a 22-gauge one-part needle, a 23-gauge butterfly needle, or a 22-gauge two-part needle. Accessing the VM is usually technically straightforward, but, in certain malformations, and particularly when under general anaesthetic, the venous spaces may empty and become challenging to access. In these cases, the use of an orthopaedic tourniquet can be used to encourage the dysplastic venous spaces to fill and become more clearly visible. Once blood is seen to drip from the needle, iodinated contrast is then injected through the needle(s) and diagnostic venography using digital subtraction angiography (DSA) is performed in order to map out the lesion and ensure there are no contraindications to proceeding to inject the sclerosant (Figure 10.9). Important information to obtain from the diagnostic venography includes intravascular location, the outflow pattern of the VM, and to ensure there is no reflux or communication with the arterial system. Once it is deemed safe to proceed, the sclerosant can be injected through the same needles using a low-dose angiographic image acquisition (Figure 10.10). This process is then repeated until there has been adequate filling of the VM or the dose limit of the sclerosing agent has been reached. All needles are then removed, and haemostasis is achieved with manual compression.

Our institutional preference for the treatment of most VMs is 3% STS. STS is typically mixed with a volume of air and contrast agent in order to make a stable foam so that the STS does not fall out of the solution. This allows it to displace blood rather than mix with it and to come into as much contact with the endothelium in the non-dependent portion of the dysplastic veins as possible. There are numerous possible compositions to form a stable foam, and the makeup of the foam is based on operator

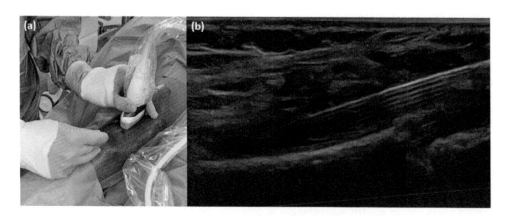

FIGURE 10.8 (a) Using a high-frequency, linear array ultrasound probe, a 22-gauge needle is used to percutaneously access the dysplastic venous spaces within a lower limb venous malformation under dynamic image guidance; (b) the ultrasound image confirms the needle tip position within the venous channel.

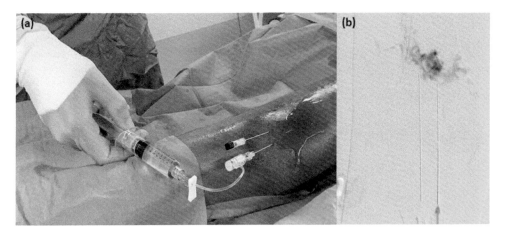

FIGURE 10.9 (a) Once the needle is confirmed to be appropriately positioned, extension tubing is attached to the needle and iodinated contrast medium is injected through the needle; (b) digital subtraction angiography is performed to map out the venous malformation.

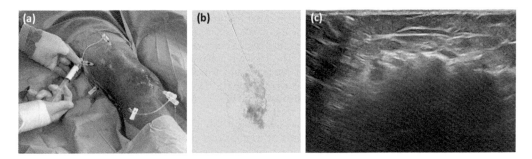

FIGURE 10.10 Once the lesion has been mapped out with contrast medium, the sclerosant, made up as a foam, is (a) injected through the same needles under (b) digital subtraction angiography; (c) following injection of the sclerosant foam, ultrasound can be performed to ensure that there has been complete filling of the venous malformation and that there are no untreated venous spaces. As the sclerosant is mixed with air, it appears hyperechoic on ultrasound and causes acoustic shadowing.

preference (Figure 10.11). The dose limit of 3% STS in a single sclerotherapy procedure is generally agreed to be 0.5 mL/kg in children and up to a maximum dose of 20 mL (11).

STS often causes significant swelling and has the potential to cause nerve injury and skin necrosis. For VMs in which this is considered to be a significant risk, such as malformations of the lips or tongue, those which involve the skin or those which are close to critical structures, such as the orbit or the airway, the operator preference may be to use bleomycin because of its more favourable profile in causing less inflammation and swelling (13). Bleomycin can be injected neat or as a foam by reconstituting it with air, Lipiodol®, and/or albumin. The recommended dose limit of bleomycin is 15,000 IU in a single treatment and can be repeated up to a maximum cumulative lifetime dose of 80,000–100,000 IU. As an aside, there is much variation in the dosage nomenclature for bleomycin (units, milligrams, and international units) and an essential need to standardise nomenclature in order to minimise the risk of prescribing errors and potential overdose (14). The maximum lifetime dose of bleomycin is primarily related to the associated risk of pulmonary fibrosis which has been reported to be up to 8% (15). The risk of lung injury is understood to be reduced by avoiding high concentrations of inspired oxygen while bleomycin is circulating systemically, so high levels of inspired oxygen should be avoided during anaesthesia. Other risks unique to bleomycin include permanent skin pigmentation resulting from inadvertent skin trauma, such as scratching or the removal of adhesive dressings, following systemic administration of bleomycin. Therefore, no adhesives, such as cannula dressings or endotracheal tube adhesives, should be used during bleomycin sclerotherapy.

VMs almost always swell following sclerotherapy, and this swelling can even be evident intraoperatively. Swelling of non-critical areas, such as the extremities, is usually well tolerated. However, swelling of VMs close to critical structures, such as the airway, can be potentially significant. An aggressive

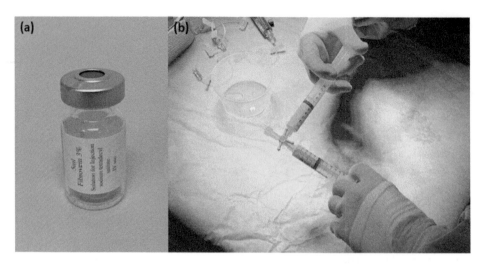

FIGURE 10.11 (a) 3% sodium tetradecyl sulfate (STS) is the most common sclerosant used; (b) it is usually made up as a foam by mixing it with iodinated contrast medium and air using two luer lock syringes and a three-way tap. The more the foam is mixed, the longer it will remain stable.

steroid regimen can be utilised intraoperatively in order to minimise the degree of post-operative swelling. Swelling is more substantial following the use of 3% STS than bleomycin.

If the treated VM is of the upper or lower limb, then a compression bandage is often applied at the end of the procedure (Figure 10.12). Patients are typically advised to leave this compression bandage in place until they can fit back into their own compression garment. The use of compression following sclerotherapy has two benefits. First, compression will retain the sclerosant in the lesion, and second, and more importantly, it will compress the treated veins and increase the likelihood of them scarring down and not refilling with blood soon after treatment.

If the injected sclerosant comes close to, or extravasates close to, the overlying skin, there is a risk of dermal injury. This is more of a risk when the VM extends into the overlying skin or in delicate areas

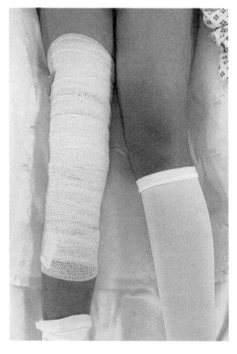

FIGURE 10.12 A compression bandage is usually applied to the treated limb – in this case, the right lower limb – after completion of the procedure and kept in place for a minimum of 24 hours. After that time, the patient is advised to remove the compression bandage and return to wearing their own compression garment.

such as the mucous membranes of the tongue or lips. Skin or mucous membrane blistering is usually minor, managed conservatively, and, with time, will heal without leaving a scar. Rarely, blistering may be so severe as to cause full thickness tissue necrosis and require plastic surgical intervention in the form of special dressings or surgical intervention and result in a scar.

If the injected sclerosant comes into contact with adjacent nerves, there is a risk of neurolysis, causing altered sensation or a motor deficit. Nerve damage is very rare and, if it occurs, is usually temporary, although it can take many months for a nerve injury to heal. Rarely, nerve injury can result in permanent disability.

STS is renally excreted, and high doses of STS can impair renal function, although usually temporarily. The risk of renal injury can be mitigated by abiding to accepted STS dose limits and ensuring the patient is very well hydrated. This may require intravenous hyperhydration of the patient before and during the procedure, especially in children who have been starved for several hours prior to anaesthesia. Most patients have dark, discoloured urine for the first few hours post-STS sclerotherapy, but this usually settles. If it does not, renal function should be actively assessed and monitored until it recovers, and this is best done under the auspices of a renal physician.

For the vast majority of VMs, multiple treatment sessions will be required. Two to three sequential courses of sclerotherapy at 4–6-week intervals are often scheduled, after which the patient is reviewed in the outpatient clinic and further sclerotherapy planned as required. A result is considered satisfactory once the symptoms have improved and are no longer considered debilitating by the patient and their family. Post-sclerotherapy imaging appearances alone should not be considered a surrogate for technical success/failure.

## SURGERY

Historically, surgical excision would be the mainstay of treatment for VM. However, the associated morbidity and the high rate of recurrence following surgical excision means that surgery is generally reserved for those VMs which have not responded to conservative measures or percutaneous sclerotherapy alone. Small VMs may be excisable, but many VMs have poorly defined margins and cross fascial planes, making complete excision challenging. VMs tend to recur if not removed completely. Patients with extensive VMs are likely to have an underlying coagulopathy, which must be actively managed around the time of any surgery by a haematologist with experience in this field.

In certain cases, in which the patient is to undergo surgical excision of a large VM and there is the potential for catastrophic intraoperative bleeding during surgical excision, the multidisciplinary team may consider preoperative embolisation of a VM immediately prior to surgical resection (16). In these cases, the VM is percutaneously accessed with a similar combination of needles as used in sclerotherapy and, following diagnostic venography to map out the malformation, a liquid embolic is injected through these needles to occlude the venous spaces (Figure 10.13). Commonly used liquid embolic agents include N-butyl cyanoacrylate glues, Onyx™, and precipitating hydrophobic injectable liquid (PHIL™). Our institutional preference is to use Histoacryl® glue, a monomeric n-butyl-2-cyanoacrylate, which polymerises and solidifies to form a cast when it comes into contact with an ionic fluid, i.e., blood. Depending on the dynamics of the VM, which can be assessed by diagnostic venography, the strength of the Histoacryl glue can be modified by diluting it with Lipiodol, an ethiodised oil which has the added benefit of being radiopaque. Transforming a VM composed of multiple venous spaces into a solid cast makes surgical resection more technically straightforward and significantly reduces the amount of intraoperative blood loss.

Surgical management of these highly varied cases can be staged or combined with sclerotherapy and embolisation and will depend on the anatomical area affected. It will, therefore, involve different specialties accordingly. Preoperative work up is imperative, often including haematology input (see Chapter 3).

## MEDICAL MANAGEMENT

Discovery of the genetic basis of VMs has enabled the use of targeted medical therapies in recent years. Sirolimus, an mTOR inhibitor, has demonstrated favourable outcomes when used in VMs that remain refractory or unsuitable for conventional therapy. Recent data suggest alpelisib, a novel selective inhibitor of p110α, the catalytic subunit of PI3K, may have a role in the treatment of VMs, including those caused by somatic *TEK* mutations, in children with a limited response to sirolimus. Further data on the long-term safety and efficacy of alpelisib in this context is needed.

# OTHER TYPES OF VENOUS ANOMALY

## VERRUCOUS VENOUS MALFORMATIONS

Verrucous VMs, previously termed verrucous haemangiomas, are a rare subtype of VM that are clinically apparent either at birth or in early childhood. They are histologically and genetically distinct from

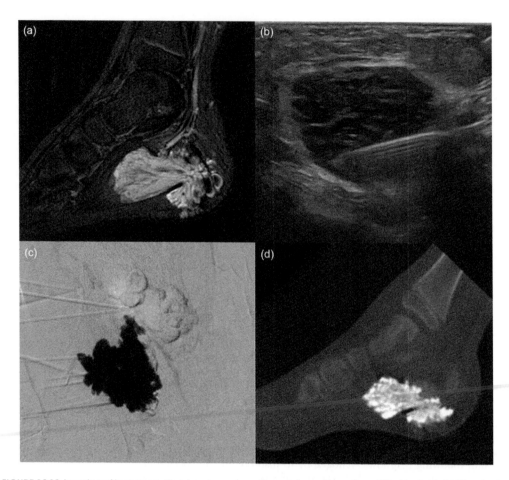

FIGURE 10.13 Imaging of teenager with a focal symptomatic venous malformation of the hindfoot. (a) T2-weighted fat-supressed sagittal MRI image demonstrates the venous malformation as a hyperintense (bright) lesion in the heel; (b) under ultrasound guidance, a 22-gauge needle is used to access the venous malformation; (c) a liquid embolic, such as Histoacryl, is injected into the malformation with the intention of filling all the venous spaces; the Lipiodol is radiopaque and is clearly seen on low-dose digital subtraction angiography; (d) cone beam CT can be performed in the IR suite to ensure complete filling of the malformation prior to transferring the patient to theatre for surgical excision of the lesion.

conventional VMs (17). Clinically, they present as solitary or multifocal deep red or purple skin stains and evolve into scaly plaques or nodules which are frequently hyperkeratotic and are occasionally painful. The clinical course can be complicated by episodes of recurrent bleeding. Histology shows immunopositivity for GLUT-1 (glucose-1-transporter), which is more commonly used as a diagnostic marker of infantile haemangiomas but can be used in this context to aid diagnosis and distinguish from classic VMs. Lesions are additionally often positive for the lymphatic endothelial cell markers podoplanin and PROX1, which can, again, help differentiate them from classic VMs (Figure 10.14). The genetic basis of verrucous VMs in 50% of cases is due to a recurrent somatic mutation in *MAP3K* (18).

The diagnosis is usually based on clinical examination (Figure 10.15) as the radiological findings can be non-specific, with ultrasound and MRI typically demonstrating multiple dilated, superficial, and deep, abnormal vessels.

Sclerotherapy does not have a role in the treatment of verrucous VMs. The treatment is complex and can often require medical, laser, and surgical interventions. Surgery may well be indicated in cases of significant and recurrent bleeding, although recurrence after surgical excision has been reported (19).

## GLOMUVENOUS MALFORMATIONS

Glomuvenous malformations are a distinct subtype of VM that are formed by an abnormal growth of blood vessels with the presence of glomus cells in the wall of the malformation. Although they can be

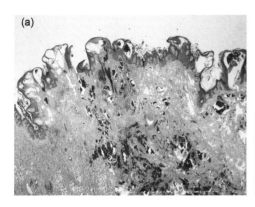
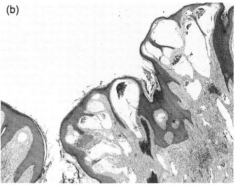

FIGURE 10.14 Photomicrographs of a verrucous vascular malformation: (a) H&E staining original magnification x12.5 and (b) H&E staining original magnification x40, with the characteristic verruciform/papillary surface architecture, dilated and abnormal lymphatic type vessels in the superficial dermis, overlying a deeper component more typical of a vascular malformation, in this example, containing predominantly abnormal capillary-type vessels.

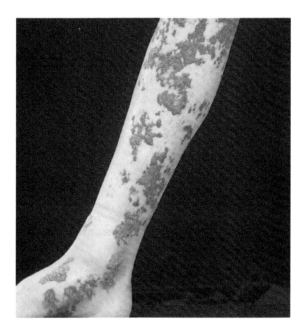

FIGURE 10.15 Typical clinical appearance of a verrucous venous malformation.

present at birth, they can present at any age and can, on occasion, be preceded by an episode of trauma. Clinically, they appear as pink/purple/blue nodules or, rarely, plaques with a characteristic cobblestone appearance and have a predilection for the extremities (Figure 10.16). They involve the skin and subcutis but can extend into deeper structures and can change over time, becoming thicker and darker in appearance. Pain is a characteristic feature of glomuvenous malformations and is exacerbated by local pressure, so compression is not a useful option for these malformations.

Imaging findings are non-specific, with ultrasound and MRI typically demonstrating dysplastic and thin-walled veins in the subcutaneous tissues. Imaging seldom confers a definitive diagnosis of a glomuvenous malformation, and, usually, a tissue diagnosis is required. However, imaging is useful in determining the anatomical extent of the malformation.

Histologically, glomuvenous malformations are characterised by the presence of pathognomonic smooth muscle-like 'glomus' cells in the media surrounding distending venous channels. Most cases of glomuvenous malformations are familial, with mutations in the glomulin GLMN gene in approximately

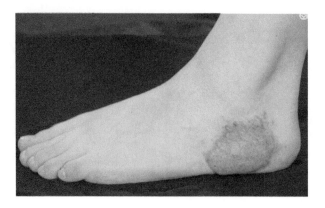

FIGURE 10.16 Typical clinical appearance of a glomuvenous malformation.

70% of cases. Germline mutations described to date are mostly small insertions and deletions with a somatic second hit observed in lesional tissue in some cases (20).

Non-surgical management with oral analgesia has been shown to reduce pain. For those malformations which do not respond to conservative measures, laser treatment with pulse-dye and Nd:YAG lasers can be considered. Depending on the anatomical location, extent, and patient's functional limitations, some glomuvenous malformations may require excision. Sclerotherapy seldom has a role in the treatment of glomuvenous malformations.

## BLUE RUBBER BLEB NAEVUS SYNDROME

Blue rubber bleb naevus syndrome (BRBNS) is a rare, multisystem, vascular disorder that is characterised by multifocal VMs which can affect any organ system but predominantly affect the skin, mucosa, and gastrointestinal tract (Figure 10.17).

BRBNS is often sporadic but can be inherited in an autosomal dominant pattern. Clinically, children present with multiple blue soft compressible cutaneous nodules at birth or in early infancy. Involvement of the skin and gastrointestinal tract is common, but involvement of all organ systems has been described including the heart, kidney, central nervous system, liver, lungs, and bladder. Cutaneous lesions are often painful, and thrombosis within lesions is common. There is significant morbidity and, rarely, mortality due to bleeding from lesions in the gastrointestinal tract, which can be evident endoscopically but is extremely challenging to manage due to the number of lesions in the gut. Excision of all gastrointestinal lesions is ambitious but is possible in experienced hands and will eradicate the risk of bleeding, as lesions do not re-grow.

Imaging, including ultrasound and MRI, show typical features of a VM. MRI is more useful in order to depict the multifocal nature of these lesions and their extent, particularly any visceral involvement. In cases of acute and clinically significant gastrointestinal bleeding, contrast enhanced CT or Technetium Tc-99m-labelled red blood cell imaging is useful to localise bleeding so that targeted endoscopic therapies can be considered.

Histopathological features of these lesions are non-specific and have overlapping features with conventional VMs. Large, dilated thin-walled vessels with a single endothelial lining are present and minimal smooth muscle may be found in the vessel walls. Calcification can also be observed within lesions (21) (Figure 10.18).

The genetic basis of BRBNS is recurrent double somatic mutations in the gene *TEK*. Mutations have been shown to be in cis, i.e., on the same allele. The mechanism behind this multifocal double somatic hit is not yet understood.

Patients with BRBNS require a multidisciplinary team approach, including surgeons, paediatrics/dermatology gastroenterology, haematology, and radiology. The mainstay of therapy in recent years has been medical management with sirolimus, which has been shown to reduce bleeding, although it is not a cure. Concurrent therapy with thalidomide in challenging cases has also been shown to decrease bleeding. Certain focal lesions may require surgical/endoscopic excision or treatment, depending on their location, extent, and the degree of pain and interference with normal function they cause.

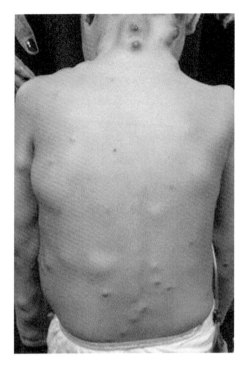

FIGURE 10.17 Typical clinical appearance of the skin lesions in blue rubber bleb naevus syndrome.

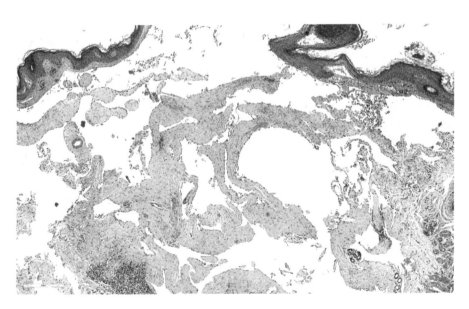

FIGURE 10.18 Photomicrograph of a superficial vascular anomaly, with normal epidermis present, composed of numerous abnormal, irregularly shaped thin-walled vascular channels lined by bland lymphatic type endothelium representing a vascular malformation, predominantly lymphatic type in this material. Original magnification x80, H&E.

## KEY MESSAGES

- VMs are benign, slow-flow, vascular malformations made up of abnormal dysplastic veins and most commonly arise due to somatic mutations.

- VMs can be focal or diffuse, occur anywhere in the body, and cross multiple anatomical territories.

- Patients most often present with symptoms of pain and swelling.

- Non-invasive imaging, including ultrasound and MRI, is usually sufficient to make a diagnosis, but, on occasion, a biopsy may be required for confirmation.

- Treatment requires a multidisciplinary team approach and can include compression garments, percutaneous sclerotherapy, and, in select cases, surgical excision.

- Percutaneous sclerotherapy is the first-line treatment option and is well tolerated. The most common sclerosing agents used are STS and bleomycin.

- There are several subtypes of VMs, including verrucous VMs, BRBNS, and glomuvenous malformations, which have special considerations.

# REFERENCES

1. Lobo-Mueller E, Amaral JG, Babyn PS, John P. Extremity vascular anomalies in children: Introduction, classification, and imaging. *Semin Musculoskelet Radiol*. 2009 Sep;13(3):210–35.
2. Nosher JL, Murillo PG, Liszewski M, Gendel V, Gribbin CE. Vascular anomalies: A pictorial review of nomenclature, diagnosis and treatment. *World J Radiol*. 2014 Sep 28;6(9):677–92.
3. Limaye N, Wouters V, Uebelhoer M, Tuominen M, Wirkkala R, Mulliken JB, et al. Somatic mutations in angiopoietin receptor gene TEK cause solitary and multiple sporadic venous malformations. *Nat Genet*. 2009 Jan;41(1):118–24.
4. Limaye N, Kangas J, Mendola A, Godfraind C, Schlögel MJ, Helaers R, et al. Somatic activating *PIK3CA* mutations cause venous malformation. *Am J Hum Genet*. 2015 Dec 3;97(6):914–21.
5. Cahill AM, Nijs ELF. Pediatric vascular malformations: Pathophysiology, diagnosis, and the role of interventional radiology. *Cardiovasc Intervent Radiol*. 2011 Aug 1;34(4):691–704.
6. Léauté-Labrèze C, Harper JI, Hoeger PH. Infantile haemangioma. *Lancet*. 2017 Jul 1;390(10089):85–94.
7. Leung M, Leung L, Fung D, Poon WL, Liu C, Chung K, et al. Management of the low-flow head and neck vascular malformations in children: The sclerotherapy protocol. *Eur J Pediatr Surg*. 2014 Feb;24(1):97–101.
8. Merrow A, Gupta A, Patel M, Adams D. 2014 Revised classification of vascular lesions from the international society for the study of vascular anomalies: Radiologic-pathologic update. *RadioGraphics*. 2016 Aug 12;36:150197.
9. Zhuo KY, Russell S, Wargon O, Adams S. Localised intravascular coagulation complicating venous malformations in children: Associations and therapeutic options. *J Paediatr Child Health*. 2017;53(8):737–41.
10. Vogelzang RL, Atassi R, Vouche M, Resnick S, Salem R. Ethanol embolotherapy of vascular malformations: Clinical outcomes at a single center. *J Vasc Interv Radiol*. 2014 Feb 1;25(2):206–13.
11. Burrows PE. Endovascular treatment of slow-flow vascular malformations. *Tech Vasc Interv Radiol*. 2013 Mar 1;16(1):12–21.
12. Chaudry G, Guevara CJ, Rialon KL, Kerr C, Mulliken JB, Greene AK, et al. Safety and efficacy of bleomycin sclerotherapy for microcystic lymphatic malformation. *Cardiovasc Intervent Radiol*. 2014 Dec 1;37(6):1476–81.
13. Horbach SER, van de Ven JS, Nieuwkerk PT, Spuls PhI, van der Horst CMAM, Reekers JA. Patient-reported outcomes of bleomycin sclerotherapy for low-flow vascular malformations and predictors of improvement. *Cardiovasc Intervent Radiol*. 2018 Oct 1;41(10):1494–1504.
14. Stefanou A, Siderov J, Society of hospital pharmacists of Australia committee of specialty practice in oncology. Medical errors. Dosage nomenclature of bleomycin needs to be standardised to avoid errors. *BMJ*. 2001 Jun 9;322(7299):1423–4.
15. Jin Y, Zou Y, Hua C, Chen H, Yang X, Ma G, et al. Treatment of early-stage extracranial arteriovenous malformations with intralesional interstitial bleomycin injection: A pilot study. *Radiology*. 2018 Apr;287(1):194–204.
16. Chewning RH, Monroe EJ, Lindberg A, Koo KSH, Ghodke BV, Gow KW, et al. Combined glue embolization and excision for the treatment of venous malformations. *CVIR Endovascular*. 2018 Oct 25;1(1):22.
17. Schmidt BAR, El Zein S, Cuoto J, Al-Ibraheemi A, Liang MG, Paltiel HJ, et al. Verrucous venous malformation-subcutaneous variant. *Am J Dermatopathol*. 2021 Dec 1;43(12):e181–4.
18. Couto JA, Vivero MP, Kozakewich HPW, Taghinia AH, Mulliken JB, Warman ML, et al. A somatic MAP3K3 mutation is associated with verrucous venous malformation. *Am J Hum Genet*. 2015 Mar 5;96(3):480–6.
19. Al-Furaih I, Al-Marzoug A, Al-Qadri N, Al-Ajlan S. Sirolimus for the management of verrucous venous malformation: A case report and literature review. *Case Rep Dermatol*. 2021;13(2):298–303.
20. Brouillard P, Boon LM, Mulliken JB, Enjolras O, Ghassibé M, Warman ML, et al. Mutations in a novel factor, Glomulin, are responsible for glomuvenous malformations ('Glomangiomas'). *Am J Hum Genet*. 2002 Apr;70(4):866–74.
21. Baigrie D, Rice AS, An IC. Blue rubber bleb nevus syndrome. In: *StatPearls* [Internet]. Treasure island (FL): StatPearls Publishing; 2022 [cited 2022 Nov 28]. Available from: http://www.ncbi.nlm.nih.gov/books/NBK541085/

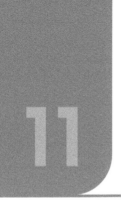

# 11 Arteriovenous Malformations

Premal A. Patel, Amir Sadri, Maanasa Polubothu, and
Neil Bulstrode

## INTRODUCTION

Arteriovenous malformations (AVMs) are high-flow lesions with arteriovenous shunting that bypasses the capillary bed. They are categorised as one of the simple vascular malformations in the International Society for the Study of Vascular Anomalies (ISSVA) classification of vascular anomalies (1). They are relatively rare but can result in significant anatomical, pathophysiological, and hemodynamic consequences and are, therefore, a potential limb or life-threatening form of vascular anomaly. Treatment is challenging and requires a multidisciplinary team (MDT) approach incorporating surgical and non-surgical interventions and, therefore, is best undertaken in high volume specialist centres.

## PATHOLOGY

AVMs are congenital vascular malformations that can be sporadic or associated with other lesions in germline syndromes. Sporadic AVM is caused by somatic activating mutations in the oncogenes *KRAS*, *BRAF* and *MAP2K1* (2). AVM can also occur as part of hereditary syndromes, in which there is typically considerable intrafamilial variability. In hereditary haemorrhagic telangiectasia (HHT), visceral AVMs (pulmonary, hepatic, cerebral) occur with cutaneous telangiectasia and epistaxis. HHT is caused by germline variants most commonly in the genes *ENG* (*HHT1*) and *ACVRL1* (*HHT2*) and rarely *SMAD4* (*HHT3*), which are inherited in an autosomal dominant manner. CM-AVM syndrome is a hereditary condition which presents with multiple capillary stains, AVM and arteriovenous fistulas, typically cutaneous or intracranial. It is caused by germline variants in the genes *RASA1* or *EPHB4* with a second somatic hit demonstrated in lesional tissue (1, 3–5). The tumour predisposition *PTEN* hamartoma tumour syndrome (PHTS) typically presents with macrocephaly, multiple hamartomas, and an increased risk of specific cancers in adulthood. PHTS is due to germline variants in the tumour suppressor gene *PTEN*, a negative regulator of the PI3K-AKT-mTOR pathway, and is inherited in an autosomal dominant manner. Patients can present with vascular anomalies including AVMs.

AVMs result from defects involving both arterial and venous vessels, resulting in direct communications between the different size vessels or a meshwork of primitive reticular networks of dysplastic minute vessels, termed the '*nidus*' (Latin for 'nest'). There is no mature capillary bed (6). There are often multiple nidi present in AVMs. Blood flow through the lesions is high-velocity flow from the arterial vasculature into the venous system due to the low resistance nature of the communications (6). AVMs undergo active angiogenesis characterised by microvascular proliferation, most prominently during adolescence, in between the otherwise mature vessels and have increased levels of pro-angiogenic factors. This process is thought to result in lesion progression (7).

## CLINICAL PRESENTATION

Sporadic AVMs present as solitary lesions. The lesions can be extensive or localised and can involve all tissue types including bone. AVMs have a persistent proliferative potential and, therefore, are seen to progress throughout life (3). The clinical presentation depends on the extent and size of the lesion and

DOI: 10.1201/9781003257417-11

can range from an asymptomatic birthmark to high-output heart failure. In some cases, AVMs can be clinically detected at birth. By puberty, around 80% of AVMs will present with symptoms or signs. They can be exacerbated during pregnancy (3, 8). A slight female preponderance has been reported (male to female ratio 1:1.5) (8).

AVMs, when superficial, initially can present as an area of pink skin discolouration and can be mistaken for a capillary malformation. As the lesion grows, there will be increased growth and warmth of the affected area. On examination, a thrill or pulsatility may be palpable, and there may be an audible bruit. Enlarged draining veins and signs of venous hypertension may be visible (Figure 11.1). If the lesion progresses and arteriovenous shunting increases, there is reduced perfusion pressure to local tissues and increased venous hypertension, resulting in tissue ischaemia, pain, ulceration and bleeding (Figure 11.2). When a large shunt is present, an AVM can cause congestive heart failure, as seen in some neonates with a vein of Galen malformation (see Chapter 14). When AVMs occur in the limbs, limb length/size discrepancy may occur. This is particularly so when the AVMs are associated with a limb overgrowth syndrome such as Parkes Weber syndrome or a RASA-1 mutation (9).

## AVM CLASSIFICATION

A number of classification systems for AVMs exist. The Schobinger classification, introduced at the 1990 meeting of the International Workshop for the Study of Vascular Anomalies in Amsterdam, is based on clinical severity and aims to provide a guide to the timing of any intervention. It outlines the clinical course of untreated AVMs from their local to eventual systemic effects and is divided into four stages (Table 11.1) (9–11).

There are two classifications describing the angioarchitecture of the AVM. The Cho classification was described in 2006 (12), and, more recently, the Yakes classification was described in 2014 (11). An angioarchitecture-based classification can help to determine the possible approaches to treatment (Table 11.2) (Figure 11.3).

# DIAGNOSTIC IMAGING

Most AVMs outside the brain can be diagnosed by clinical assessment and patient history (13). This initial assessment should be supplemented by Duplex ultrasound. Other investigations, such as magnetic resonance imaging (MRI), MR angiography (MRA), computerised tomography (CT), and CT angiography (CTA), may also help provide additional information, but angiography is the gold standard imaging modality for AVMs and is required for planning any subsequent treatment (Figures 11.1, 11.4, 11.5).

## ULTRASOUND

On ultrasound imaging, the lesion will be composed of a conglomerate of tortuous vessels with no discrete soft tissue mass. However, some AVMs demonstrate no abnormality on greyscale imaging (14). The presence of a soft tissue mass indicates an alternative diagnosis such as a vascular tumour. There may sometimes be thickening or altered echogenicity of the soft tissues around an AVM due to oedema or fibro-fatty infiltration (15). Colour Doppler ultrasound shows a high-flow hypervascular lesion with a high vessel density with multidirectional flow (Figures 11.4 and 11.5). Doppler waveforms in the feeding arteries show high velocities with low resistance waveforms and spectral broadening. Aliasing and turbulent flow is seen at the region of the nidus in keeping with very fast flow. Identification of these areas can help target direct punctures during interventions (9). In the venous outflow, turbulent arterialised flow is seen (14).

## MRI

MR imaging is often the preferred imaging modality to determine the extent of an AVM and its relationship to adjacent structures. MRA can be used to give detail about arterial inflow, the nidus, and the venous outflow. The degree of soft tissue and bone involvement can be assessed. Areas of thrombosis in the lesion can be detected as can complications such as infection, haemorrhage, or ischaemia. Dynamic time-resolved MRA can help assess flow dynamics with the identification of a vascular nidus (Figure 11.3) (16).

## CT

Some teams prefer CTA as the cross-sectional imaging modality for AVMs. CT is most useful for AVMs that have bony involvement and lesions that have dilated veins or venous aneurysms (17).

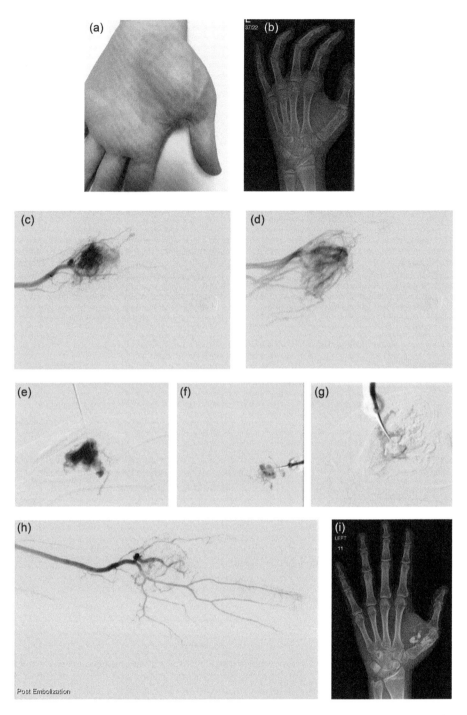

FIGURE 11.1 Teenager with painful AVM of the hand. A clinical photograph (a) of the palmar surface of the hand shows pink skin discolouration and enlarged superficial veins. Hand radiograph (b) shows erosion of the first metacarpal bone due to an intraosseous AVM. Images from an angiogram of the hand early in the arterial phase (c) and later in the arterial phase (d) delineate the complex AVM with no clearly defined feeding arteries. There is shunting to multiple outflow veins and poor distal perfusion of the normal digital arteries. Embolisation (e, f, and g) was performed with Histoacryl glue diluted and opacified with Lipiodol (ethiodised oil) using a direct puncture approach three times over the course of 4 months. The embolisation images demonstrate occlusion of the venous outflow and arterial inflow, thus, obliterating the nidus. The final angiogram image (h) shows almost no AVM with significant improvement in perfusion of distal normal tissues. Follow-up hand radiograph (i) shows embolic material in the thenar space and in the first metacarpal bone.

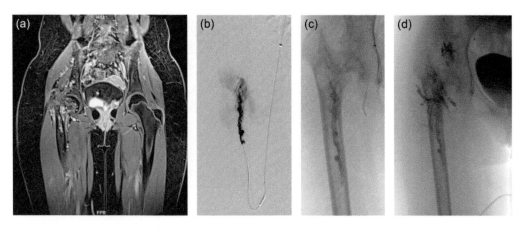

FIGURE 11.2 Teenager with an AVM of the hip with symptoms of claudication in the lower limb due to vascular steal. Coronal post-contrast fat-saturated T1-weighted MRI (a) shows numerous enhancing vessels around the right hip and in the femur and iliac bone. The femoral neck and head are deformed due to avascular necrosis secondary to the local vascular steal phenomenon. An image from a superselective angiogram of one of the arterial feeding vessels in the femur (b) confirms the vessel to be large and tortuous; shunting to large veins is seen. This vessel was embolised with PHIL™, and post-embolisation fluoroscopy (c) shows the embolic material cast has penetrated deep into the lesion. Embolisation was performed from two further arterial feeding vessels. Fluoroscopic image at completion (d) shows complete embolisation of the AVM including the intra-osseous components in the femur and iliac bone.

**TABLE 11.1**  Schobinger clinical classification of AVMs

| Schobinger Classification | Stage | Clinical Features |
|---|---|---|
| Stage I | Quiescence | Cutaneous blush, skin warmth, and arteriovenous shunt on Doppler ultrasound, the AVM causes no clinical symptoms |
| Stage II | Expansion | Darkening blush, the lesion shows pulsation has a palpable thrill, audible bruit, and enlarged arterialised tortuous/tense veins |
| Stage III | Destruction | Steal, distal ischemia, pain, dystrophic skin changes, ulceration which can be non-healing and necrosis with soft tissue and bony changes |
| Stage IV | Decompensation | Features of Stage III with the addition of high-output cardiac failure |

*Source:* Adapted from [9–11].

## ANGIOGRAPHY

Catheter angiography is mandatory before any therapeutic interventions and is usually best performed by the team who will be performing any definitive intervention. It allows precise evaluation of the feeding arteries and draining veins of the malformation and an assessment of the feasibility of embolisation and surgery. The angiographic characteristics of AVMs are dilatation and lengthening of afferent arteries, with early opacification of enlarged veins. Angiography should involve non-selective acquisitions to provide an overview of arterial feeding vessels and venous drainage (Figure 11.4). Then, selective and super-selective catheterisations are necessary to assess for nidi and to plan treatment. Due to the fast flow nature of AVMs, high frame rate digital subtraction angiography (DSA) should be performed.

## ADDITIONAL IMAGING

Plain radiographs are generally not useful except to monitor the effects of AVMs on bones (Figure 11.1). Patients with an AVM should have an echocardiogram, in particular before any intervention, to assess for any early signs of heart failure.

**TABLE 11.2** Yakes classification of AVM angioarchitecture

| Yakes Type | Angioarchitecture |
|---|---|
| Type I | Direct artery/arteriole to vein/venule connection. |
| Type II | Multiple inflow arteries/arterioles connecting through an intervening 'nidus' without any intervening capillary beds draining into multiple outflow veins. |
| Type IIIa | Multiple inflow arterioles shunting into an aneurysmal vein that has a single vein outflow. The fistulae are in the vein wall. |
| Type IIIb | Multiple inflow arterioles shunting into an aneurysmal vein with multiple outflow veins. The fistulae are in the vein wall. |
| Type IV | Multiple arteries/arterioles forming innumerable microfistulae that diffusely infiltrate the affected tissue. Capillary beds are also present among the innumerable arterio-venous fistulae (AVFs) and maintain local tissue viability. The innumerable micro-AVFs drain blood at near-arterial pressure into multiple veins. The tissue's normal post-capillary venous drainage then competes with the arterialised vein outflow for drainage, causing venous hypertension in the affected tissue. |

*Source:* Adapted from [9–11].

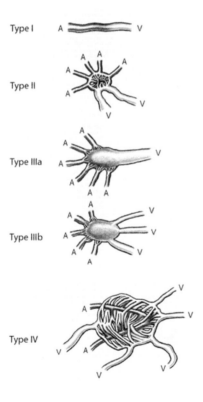

FIGURE 11.3 Schematic diagrams demonstrating Yakes AVM angioarchitecture classification. (Adapted from [11].)

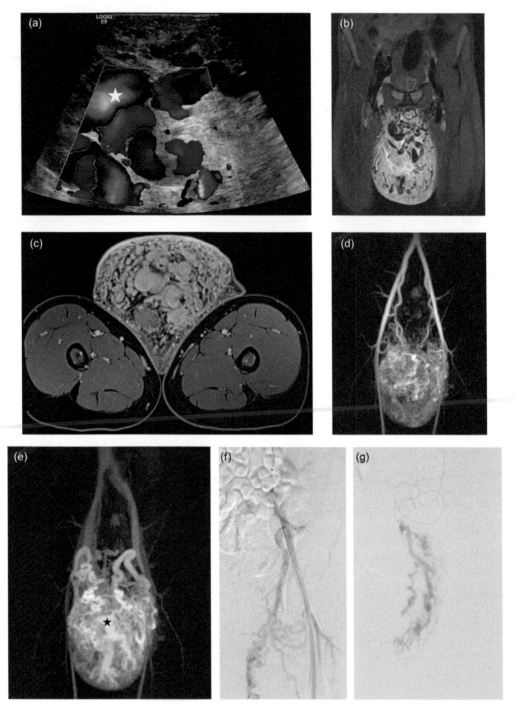

FIGURE 11.4 Teenager with large scrotal AVM with ischaemic skin necrosis. Ultrasound (a) demonstrating high vessel density with large venous spaces. Coronal short tau inversion recovery MRI (b) demonstrates a large AVM with multiple flow voids. Post-contrast T1-weighted fat-saturated axial MRI (c) shows enhancement of numerous vessels. The right testis is surrounded by the AVM. Time-resolved MRA in the early arterial phase (d) shows tortuous arterial feeders to the complex AVM, and a late arterial image (e) shows filling of large venous spaces in the lesion and early filling of dilated outflow veins. Angiogram from the left common iliac artery (f) demonstrates some of the tortuous hypertrophied arterial feeders to the AVM. A superselective angiogram (g) demonstrates tortuous feeding arteries. Note the multiple loops in the microcatheter required to reach a distal position. A relatively proximal preoperative embolisation was performed with Histoacryl glue. The post-embolisation angiogram (h) shows no filling from the embolised component of the AVM, with the glue cast visible. A fluoroscopic image (i) shows extensive glue cast, and the completion angiogram (j) shows no shunting through the AVM. The patient underwent resection of the AVM the day after embolisation. Follow-up ultrasound (k) shows testes with minimal residual AVM.

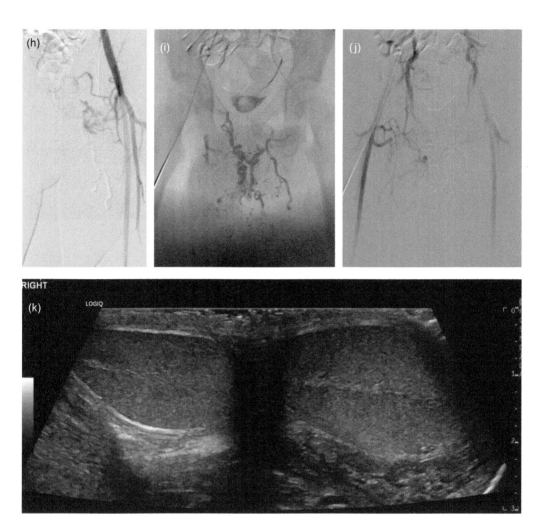

FIGURE 11.4 Continued.

## HISTOPATHOLOGY

AVMs are usually diagnosed on clinical and radiological features, and histopathology is less useful. Histological findings may be variable depending on site, chronicity, and previous therapy attempts. The characteristic features are abnormal muscular vessels, including abnormal arteries, large and thick-walled 'arterisalised' veins, and other vascular structures admixed, including veins and lymphatics. Arteries may be structurally abnormal with disruption of the internal elastic lamina and transition to indeterminate morphology, with vessels resembling hypertensive veins. These veins may show thickening of the muscular layer and chronic fibrosis. There are no specific immunohistochemical markers of AVMs, but special stains such as elastin van Giesen may be useful to highlight the vascular anatomy and especially the elastic lamina (Figure 11.6).

## TREATMENT

Embolisation or embolisation in combination with surgery are the main treatments for AVMs but are associated with a significant risk of complications and morbidity. Indications for treatment are cardiac failure and effects of ischaemia, such as skin ulceration, bleeding, and pain. Asymptomatic (Schobinger Stage I) lesions should be left alone. Treatment should be offered for Schobinger Stage III and IV lesions and for Stage II, which are rapidly expanding. The aims of treatment are to reduce pain, improve functional impairment, and improve cardiac failure if present. Treatment can be done with the aim of being curative or palliative, depending on the anatomy and extent of the AVM. Localised lesions may be better treated by surgical resection, which has a lower recurrence rate and longer time to recurrence

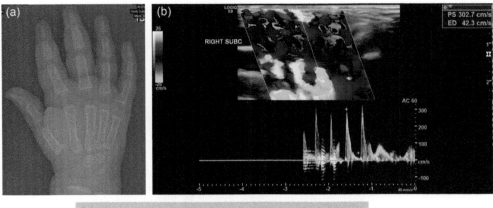

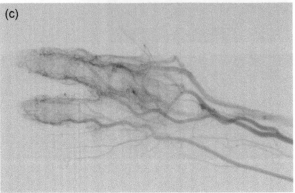

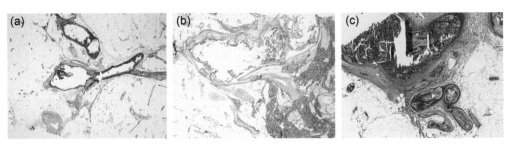

FIGURE 11.5 Toddler with an asymptomatic AVM of the hand affecting the digits. Radiograph (a) shows thickening of soft tissue of the index and middle finger. Colour Doppler ultrasound (b) shows a lesion with fast multidirectional flow. Angiography (c) shows tortuous hypertrophied arterial supply to the lesion with rapid shunting to the outflow veins via innumerable tiny fistulas.

than embolisation (18). Diffuse lesions are better treated by embolisation with a palliative symptom control goal. Generally, AVMs are considered challenging lesions to manage with high recurrence rates following treatment. In a series of 272 patients, the recurrence rate within one year after resection (with or without embolisation) was 57% and 86% with embolisation alone (18).

## EMBOLISATION

### Technique

Angiography and embolisation can be performed in the same sitting or as two separate procedures, which provides time for planning and MDT discussion regarding combined approaches. The aim of embolisation is to eliminate the AVM nidi. Embolisation of feeding arteries, which leaves the nidus intact, may, instead, result in proliferation of the lesion (6). A symptom-based approach is also required.

FIGURE 11.6 Photomicrographs of a vascular lesion demonstrating large abnormal vessels, including arteries, veins, and abnormal 'arterialised' veins with thick walls. (a) H&E original magnification x40 and (b) x100. The features are highlighted with van Giesen staining (c) (original magnification x100), which also more clearly illustrates the intraluminal material secondary to therapy.

Reduction of inflow should be an aim when there is bleeding and pain thought to be secondary to venous hypertension. If there is skin destruction due to ischaemia, the aim should be to reduce the steal phenomenon (17). When the AVMs are extensive, nidi in the region of symptoms should be targeted. Lesions often progress following embolisation; therefore, it may be helpful to explain to patients to think of embolisation as a method of lesion 'control' rather than 'cure'.

The embolisation approach will vary depending on the AVM angioarchitecture. The most common approach is transarterial, selective microcatheter embolisation of each feeding vessel with the aim of treating the nidus, the inflow and the outflow vessels. A transvenous approach is useful when numerous arterial feeders reach one fistula point with one venous drainage (Yakes Type IIIa). Direct puncture of the nidus with or without occlusion of the draining vein can also be used (Figure 11.1).

Angiography and embolisation is performed under general anaesthesia due to the length of the procedure and the pain which can occur during embolisation and to provide a motionless target. Arterial access is achieved under ultrasound guidance, usually a common femoral artery. The smallest sheath size possible should be used; generally a 4 Fr sheath is sufficient for a triaxial system (sheath, 4 Fr guide catheter, and a smaller microcatheter). Thin-walled, low profile sheaths designed for radial access can be used in children's common femoral arteries, allowing a smaller access site and ensuring that less arterial lumen is occupied for the duration of the procedure. It is recommended that for children <15 kg, continuous sheath flush is achieved using a pressurised saline drip bag attached to the sidearm of the vascular sheath as thrombotic complications of arterial access are higher in children than in adults (19). Radiation dose reduction measures should be strongly considered, such as removal of the grid, maximising the air gap, reducing fluoroscopy pulse rate and collimating to the area of interest when performing angiography in children.

When performing embolisation, superselective catheter placement is essential. Immediately prior to embolisation, DSA from the intended embolisation point should be performed to assess the anticipated distribution of the embolic agent. Speed of flow through the nidus can be assessed. If the flow is too fast to allow safe embolisation, it can be slowed by the use of a tourniquet or balloon occlusion of arterial inflow or venous outflow. If it is not possible to reach the AVM nidus with an endovascular approach, direct percutaneous puncture techniques should be considered. Direct punctures are usually performed with 21–23G needles under ultrasound guidance. Careful angiography through the needles should be performed prior to embolisation. Embolisation should be performed with continuous fluoroscopic imaging to monitor the antegrade progress of embolic material and to detect whether reflux is occurring. Following embolic injections, a repeat DSA is performed to assess for vessel closure and look for any non-target embolisation (Figures 11.1, 11.3 and 11.4).

On arterial sheath removal, haemostasis should be ensured by gentle manual compression. Use of arterial closure devices in children is not recommended. Bed rest is recommended for at least 4 hours to protect the arterial access site. Following embolisation, children usually require at least an overnight admission to manage pain and assess the effects of any local swelling.

## Embolic Agents

Embolic agents used for AVM embolisation are generally permanent agents. Embolic agents can be liquid, such as ethanol, glue or Onyx™, or mechanical products such as coils. Particles should not be used, as they are highly likely to flow through the shunts and cause unintended embolisation elsewhere, such as the lungs or brain.

Liquid agents progress through the lesion on injection and, therefore, are more likely to reach all the way to the nidus. They carry less recanalisation risk than mechanical agents. Ethanol is the agent of choice for some interventional radiologists, as it causes endothelial ablation (17). However, it can cause spasm in the pulmonary arteries, causing right ventricular strain and vascular collapse (9), and non-target embolisation can result in widespread ischaemia. Use of ethanol for AVM embolisation, thus, requires extensive training and sufficient experience to minimise complications. Glues, such as Histoacryl® and Glubran® 2, polymerise on contact with ionic substances such as blood. They are diluted and opacified with Lipiodol (ethiodised oil) prior to injection to help achieve nidal penetration (Figure 11.1). Non-adhesive liquid embolic agents such as Onyx™ and PHIL™ harden from the outside in, also allowing deep penetration of the lesion (Figure 11.4).

Embolisation coils are soft metal coils which can cause mechanical vessel occlusion if densely packed or thrombotic occlusion by slowing flow. Coils are generally not a first-line embolic material for AVMs, as they would result in too proximal an arterial closure. However, nidal closure can be achieved in some cases by deploying coils on the venous side of the shunt (20).

## Risks

The risks of embolisation can be thought of as non-target embolisation. There can be unwanted venous occlusion or passage of embolic material to the pulmonary circulation if liquid agents are injected too quickly or are prepared such that they travel through the nidus without setting. Similarly, embolic agents can reflux back along the injected vessel and into non-AVM supplying branches and can result in tissue ischaemia and necrosis at unintended, distant sites, including skin, muscle, and nerves. Embolisation of feeding arteries too proximally (without treatment of the nidus) simply results in angiogenesis and revascularisation of the AVM with small, more tortuous vessels which are far more difficult to treat.

## CRYOABLATION

Cryoablation is a thermal ablation modality which involves freezing tissues to kill them. It has been successfully used for some vascular anomalies which are resistant to traditional treatments, such as fibro-adipose vascular anomalies (21). Cryoablation for residual AVMs, post-embolisation, has been reported in a series of four patients with complete nidal obliteration in 75% of cases but with a 75% complication rate (22). Therefore, at present, ablation is not a standard treatment modality for these lesions but may be used more frequently in the future.

## BLEOMYCIN SCLEROTHERAPY

Bleomycin sclerotherapy is known to be effective in reducing the size and symptoms of low-flow vascular malformations with lower adverse event rates and fewer severe complications than other sclerosants (23). Intralesional interstitial bleomycin injection to treat early-stage (Schobinger Stage I or II) extracranial AVMs has been reported in a series of 34 patients with 84% of cases showing response, including 28% in whom there was complete response. This may be a treatment which is used more frequently in the future, possibly as an adjunct to embolisation.

## SURGERY

Surgical resection of AVMs should be considered for patients with localised disease. Surgery can be combined with presurgical embolisation to reduce intraoperative bleeding, but embolisation does not reduce the volume of tissue resected. When preceded by embolisation, surgery should happen within 2–3 days of preoperative embolisation (Figures 11.7 and 11.8). Caution should be taken with a surgical approach, as AVMs are known to respond to surgical trauma by progression, resulting in high post-surgical 'recurrence' rates if not completely excised. Amputation should be considered for extremity AVMs causing life or limb-threatening symptoms.

Preoperative imaging of the AVM should be analysed to determine whether the tumour is confined to a specific compartment or tissue plane. If the AVM does not cross the deep fascia, surgical resection is safest by starting the excision within normal tissue and circumscribing the AVM. This allows dissection within normal tissue and, thus, reduces the intraoperative blood loss. Nevertheless, feeding vessels are inevitably encountered and either cauterised or ligated.

If the AVM invades the deep fascia and enters muscle compartments, a decision has to be made as to whether muscle can be sacrificed without compromising function. Again, excision through normal tissue is preferable, as this reduces blood loss. However, in some circumstances, disease may not be fully resectable. This makes vascular control intraoperatively more challenging. In these situations, it is best to resect with two first surgeons and many assistants. One surgeon excises, while the other achieves haemostasis. Suture ligation with quilting sutures, adrenaline, and tranexamic acid-soaked gauze are usually required. In some cases, resection is paused while the anaesthetic team replaces blood loss and maintains the patient's blood pressure.

Once the AVM has been resected and haemostasis achieved, surgical reconstruction of the area begins. In some cases, direct closure of wound edges can be achieved. If this is not possible, local flap options are considered. If the wound bed has sufficient vascularity with no exposed bone, tendon, or dura, then a skin graft can be applied to the wound. In rare circumstances, complex-free tissue transfer with microvascular reconstruction is needed (24).

## MEDICAL MANAGEMENT

Currently there are no medications approved for the treatment of AVMs. However, recent advances in understanding the genetic basis of AVM present a possible therapeutic strategy with repurposing of cancer therapies for sporadic AVM caused by hotspot mutations in common oncogenes *KRAS*, *BRAF*, and *MAP2K1*. MEK inhibition has shown efficacy in AVM preclinical studies and animal models. Trametinib, a selective MEK1/MEK2 inhibitor, has shown promise in two recent cases of a *KRAS* and *MAP2K1* AVM (25, 26) with objective decrease in AVM size within 6 months of initiation with no significant adverse effects (3). Recent evidence also suggests a role for thalidomide, an anti-angiogenic agent used previously to manage gastrointestinal bleeding in vascular malformations, to improve chronic pain, bleeding, and ulceration in adult AVM, although it must be noted the side effect profile

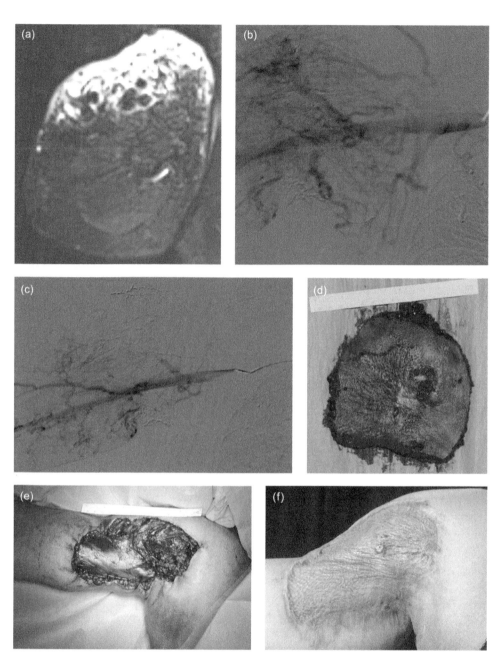

FIGURE 11.7 Teenager with symptomatic AVM of the upper limb and chest wall. Nine embolisations, starting at 4 years of age, had been performed using a combination of Onyx™ and Histoacryl®, using arterial and transvenous approaches. Over the preceding 2 years, the patient had been suffering pain, recurrent bleeding, and ulceration of the component on the upper arm. Axial T2-weighted fat-suppressed MRI (a) demonstrates large vessels in the superficial soft tissues of the arm with high signal in the intervening tissue consistent with oedema. Angiogram prior to preoperative embolisation (b) shows numerous arteriovenous shunts in the area of ulceration. Embolisation from five arterial feeders was performed with Histoacryl. Completion angiography (c) shows markedly less vascularity in the area to be resected. Intraoperative photograph of the skin surface of the resected tissue (d) showing the area of skin necrosis and scar from repeated ulceration, and an intraoperative photograph of the resection bed (e) shows resection of the subcutaneous tissue down to muscle with satisfactory haemostasis. This surgical site was covered with a split-thickness skin graft (f).

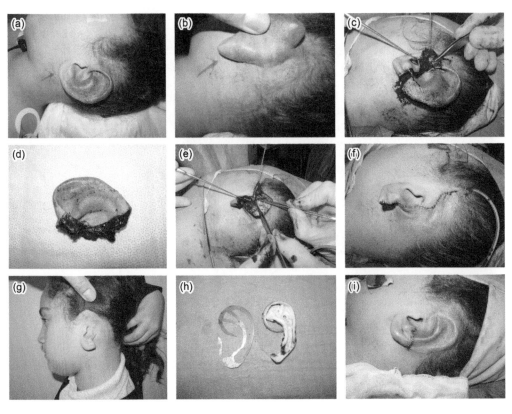

FIGURE 11.8 A 9-year-old girl with a Type 2 AVM of the ear (see [24] for classification) affecting the superior two-thirds of the ear with lobular and tragal sparing, anterior view (a), posterior view (b), with discoloration post-embolisation performed one day prior to surgical excision, as described in (24). Intraoperative views (c) demonstrating the main feeding artery, the partially resected ear (d), and the intact superficial temporal vessels after resection (e). The post-resection view with spared lobule and tragus (f). Twelve months post-resection clinical view demonstrating no recurrence or progression (g). The carved rib cartilage framework (h) and post-first stage of the ear reconstruction process (i).

is significant, and this should be used cautiously by experienced providers (27). A medical management approach to AVMs may be useful in cases in which angioarchitecture precludes embolisation and soft tissue location precludes limb-sparing surgery. Clinical trials are needed to evaluate the safety and efficacy of these targeted therapies in clinical practice.

## KEY MESSAGES

- AVMs are lesions in which there is arteriovenous shunting through a 'nidus' without an intervening capillary bed.

- AVMs are classified according to symptoms and angiographic appearances.

- Clinical assessment and ultrasound are often sufficient to make a diagnosis. MRI can provide information regarding the distribution of the lesion, and angiography is used to plan treatment.

- AVMs are difficult to manage and are best managed by a multidisciplinary approach in a high-volume centre.

- Treatment options include embolisation and surgery. Medical management options based on genetic mutations are increasing.

Arteriovenous Malformations

# REFERENCES

1. International Society for the Study of Vascular Anomalies. ISSVA Classification of Vascular Anomalies 2023. [Internet] [cited 2023]. Available from http://issva.org/classification
2. Al-Olabi L, Polubothu S, Dowsett K, et al. (2018) Mosaic RAS/MAPK variants cause sporadic vascular malformations which respond to targeted therapy. *J Clin Invest* 128:1496–1508. https://doi.org/10.1172/JCI98589
3. Schimmel K, Ali MK, Tan SY, et al. (2021) Arteriovenous malformations – current understanding of the pathogenesis with implications for treatment. *Int J Mol Sci* 22:9037. https://doi.org/10.3390/ijms22169037
4. Eerola I, Boon LM, Mulliken JB, et al. (2003) Capillary malformation-arteriovenous malformation, a new clinical and genetic disorder caused by RASA1 mutations. *Am J Hum Genet* 73:1240–1249. https://doi.org/10.1086/379793
5. Amyere M, Revencu N, Helaers R, et al. (2017) Germline loss-of-function mutations in EPHB4 cause a second form of capillary malformation–arteriovenous malformation (CM-AVM2) deregulating RAS-MAPK signaling. *Circulation* 136:1037–1048. https://doi.org/10.1161/CIRCULATIONAHA.116.026886
6. Lee BB, Baumgartner I, Berlien HP, et al. (2013) Consensus document of the International Union of Angiology (IUA)-2013. Current concept on the management of arterio-venous management. *Int Angiol J Int Union Angiol* 32:9–36.
7. Utami AM, Azahaf S, de Boer OJ, et al. (2021) A literature review of microvascular proliferation in arteriovenous malformations of skin and soft tissue. *J Clin Transl Res* 7:540–557.
8. Kohout MP, Hansen M, Pribaz JJ, Mulliken JB. (1998) Arteriovenous malformations of the head and neck: Natural history and management. *Plast Reconstr Surg* 102:643–654. https://doi.org/10.1097/00006534-199809030-00006
9. Soulez G, Gilbert, MD, FRCPC, P, Giroux, MD, FRCPC, M-F, et al. (2019) Interventional management of arteriovenous malformations. *Tech Vasc Interv Radiol* 22:100633. https://doi.org/10.1016/j.tvir.2019.100633
10. Legiehn GM, Heran MKS. (2006) Classification, diagnosis, and interventional radiologic management of vascular malformations. *Orthop Clin North Am* 37:435–474, vii–viii. https://doi.org/10.1016/j.ocl.2006.04.005
11. Yakes W, Baumgartner. I. (2014) Interventional treatment of arterio-venous malformations. Gefässchirurgie 19:325–330. https://doi.org/10.1007/s00772-013-1303-9
12. Cho SK, Do YS, Shin SW, et al. (2006) Arteriovenous malformations of the body and extremities: Analysis of therapeutic outcomes and approaches according to a modified angiographic classification. *J Endovasc Ther Off J Int Soc Endovasc Spec* 13:527–538. https://doi.org/10.1583/05-1769.1
13. Clemens RK, Pfammatter T, Meier TO, et al. (2015) Combined and complex vascular malformations. *VASA Z Gefasskrankheiten* 44:92–105. https://doi.org/10.1024/0301-1526/a000414
14. Johnson CM, Navarro OM. (2017) Clinical and sonographic features of pediatric soft-tissue vascular anomalies part 2: Vascular malformations. *Pediatr Radiol* 47:1196–1208. https://doi.org/10.1007/s00247-017-3906-x
15. Dubois J, Alison M. (2010) Vascular anomalies: What a radiologist needs to know. *Pediatr Radiol* 40:895–905. https://doi.org/10.1007/s00247-010-1621-y
16. Dunham GM, Ingraham CR, Maki JH, Vaidya SS. (2016) Finding the nidus: Detection and workup of non–central nervous system arteriovenous malformations. *RadioGraphics* 36:891–903. https://doi.org/10.1148/rg.2016150177
17. Gilbert P, Dubois J, Giroux MF, Soulez G. (2017) New treatment approaches to arteriovenous malformations. *Semin Interv Radiol* 34:258–271. https://doi.org/10.1055/s-0037-1604299
18. Liu AS, Mulliken JB, Zurakowski D, et al. (2010) Extracranial arteriovenous malformations: Natural progression and recurrence after treatment. *Plast Reconstr Surg* 125:1185–1194. https://doi.org/10.1097/PRS.0b013e3181d18070
19. Heran MKS, Marshalleck F, Temple M, et al. (2010) Joint quality improvement guidelines for pediatric arterial access and arteriography: From the Societies of Interventional Radiology and Pediatric Radiology. *J Vasc Interv Radiol JVIR* 21:32–43. https://doi.org/10.1016/j.jvir.2009.09.006
20. Jackson JE, Mansfield AO, Allison DJ. (1996) Treatment of high-flow vascular malformations by venous embolization aided by flow occlusion techniques. *Cardiovasc Intervent Radiol* 19:323–328. https://doi.org/10.1007/BF02570183
21. Shaikh R. (2017) Percutaneous image-guided cryoablation in vascular anomalies. *Semin Interv Radiol* 34:280–287. https://doi.org/10.1055/s-0037-1604453
22. Woolen S, Gemmete JJ. (2016) Treatment of residual facial arteriovenous malformations after embolization with percutaneous cryotherapy. *J Vasc Interv Radiol JVIR* 27:1570–1575. https://doi.org/10.1016/j.jvir.2016.05.027
23. Horbach SER, Rigter IM, Smitt JHS, et al. (2016) Intralesional bleomycin injections for vascular malformations: A systematic review and meta-analysis. *Plast Reconstr Surg* 137:244–256. https://doi.org/10.1097/PRS.0000000000001924
24. Bulstrode NW, Lese I, Aldabbas M, et al. (2021) Arterio-venous malformations of the ear: Description of distinct anatomical presentation and multidisciplinary management approach. *J Plast Reconstr Aesthetic Surg JPRAS* 74:1574–1581. https://doi.org/10.1016/j.bjps.2020.11.018
25. Edwards EA, Phelps AS, Cooke D, et al. (2020) Monitoring arteriovenous malformation response to genotype-targeted therapy. *Pediatrics* 146:e20193206. https://doi.org/10.1542/peds.2019-3206
26. Lekwuttikarn R, Lim YH, Admani S, et al. (2019) Genotype-guided medical treatment of an arteriovenous malformation in a child. *JAMA Dermatol* 155:256–257. https://doi.org/10.1001/jamadermatol.2018.4653
27. Boone LM, Dekeuleneer V, Coulie J, et al. (2022) Case report study of thalidomide therapy in 18 patients with severe arteriovenous malformations. *Nat Cardiovasc Res* 1:562–567.

# Complex Vascular Anomalies and Overgrowth Syndromes

12

Bran Sivakumar, Matthew Lloyd Jones, Deborah Eastwood, and Maanasa Polubothu

## INTRODUCTION

Complex vascular anomalies and overgrowth syndromes are a clinically heterogenous group. Historically, various monikers were used to describe different complex vascular anomalies and overgrowth syndromes with overlapping clinical features. The discovery of the genetic basis of this diverse spectrum of conditions has enabled refined stratification of these cohorts. Establishing the underlying genetic basis has given insights into the molecular mechanisms leading to disease and allowed us to group many clinically delineated syndromes, previously thought to be disparate, based primarily on their causative genetic mutation. In addition, knowledge of the underlying genetics has enabled the development of targeted medical therapies for these cohorts. However, phenotypic discrimination of these disorders plays a pivotal role in the diagnosis and management, as entirely different phenotypes can be caused by similar genetic variants. Conversely, the reverse is also true; different genotypes may manifest with similar phenotypical traits. Recognising classic clinical features and associations is still extremely important to inform prognosis, help direct genetic testing, channel referrals to relevant specialists, and steer medical and surgical management. Therefore, a multi-disciplinary team approach is extremely important in managing patients with these multi-faceted and complex pathologies.

## CLINICAL PRESENTATION

### PIK3CA-RELATED OVERGROWTH SPECTRUM

*PIK3CA*-related overgrowth spectrum (PROS) is an umbrella term used to incorporate a collection of conditions that can, in some cases, be caused by mosaicism for somatic activating mutations in the gene *PIK3CA* (1). These are clinically delineated conditions and range from syndromes of severe overgrowth with associated complex vascular anomalies to more simple lesions, such as isolated venous malformations, or isolated macrodactyly. As with all mosaic conditions, the phenotype depends on both the timing of the mutation in fetal development and the cell type in which the mutation occurs, with more extensive phenotypes believed to be due to an early somatic mutation. In addition to isolated vascular anomalies and isolated overgrowth, the spectrum of PROS includes several complex clinically defined syndromes such as megalencephaly-capillary malformation syndrome, Congenital lipomatous overgrowth, vascular malformation, epidermal naevi, scoliosis/skeletal anomalies (CLOVES) syndrome, Klippel–Trénaunay syndrome, and aberrant muscle syndrome. PROS has been associated with an increased risk of Wilms' tumour, though the incidence of the tumour in this cohort is low. Recent international Wilms' tumour consensus guidelines suggest imaging surveillance is not necessary in this patient cohort (2). Clinicians still may prefer to adopt a 6–12 monthly surveillance protocol with abdominal ultrasounds in the most extensive phenotypes until the age of 7 years. Complex syndromes associated with PROS are discussed in more detail below.

### MEGALENCEPHALY-CAPILLARY MALFORMATION SYNDROME

Megalencephaly-capillary malformation syndrome (MCAP; MIM 602501) manifests with overgrowth of the brain and somatic tissues. This disorder classically presents with congenital hemimegalencephaly

DOI: 10.1201/9781003257417-12

or megalencephaly (occipitofrontal circumference [OFC] ≥ 3 SD). Neurological symptoms can be mild with the most severely affected cases presenting with seizures, hypotonia, and intellectual disability. Classic magnetic resonance imaging (MRI) findings in this cohort include megalencephaly or hemimegalencephaly, polymicrogyria, and a thickened corpus callosum. Characteristic cutaneous findings include persistent midline facial nevus simplex/capillary malformation and generalised reticulate capillary malformations which can affect the face, trunk, and limbs.

## CLOVES SYNDROME

Congenital lipomatous overgrowth, vascular malformation, epidermal naevi, scoliosis/skeletal anomalies (CLOVES) have characteristic features which include congenital asymmetric lipomatous overgrowth of the trunk, causing progressive scoliosis when infiltrating adjacent tissues. The truncal lipomatous masses may contain a variable portion of lymphatic malformation. Overlying mixed slow-flow vascular malformations are very common, although spinal and paraspinal arteriovenous malformations (AVMs) have also been described. Epidermal naevi are common and can be subtle. Musculoskeletal anomalies most commonly affect the feet and hands and include wide hands and feet, macrodactyly, and a wide sandal gap.

## KLIPPEL–TRÉNAUNAY SYNDROME

Klippel–Trénaunay syndrome (KTS) is traditionally defined by the presence of a capillary malformation, venous malformation, and limb overgrowth with or without a lymphatic malformation (3) (Figure 12.1). Typically, the features are confined to the lower limb; however, it can rarely present with unilateral upper limb overgrowth. Soft tissue overgrowth is predominantly fatty and centred within extrafascial/subcutaneous compartments. Osseous overgrowth commonly follows the soft tissue overgrowth. The capillary malformation may present with vesicles suggestive of an underlying lymphatic component. Lymphatic malformations can be of the macrocystic, microcystic, or combined types and present with pain and recurrent infections. A persistent embryonic vein, also known as the lateral marginal vein or vein of Servelle, is present in the affected limb in 70% of patients. Awareness of these anomalous venous channels is vital in patients with complex overgrowth because they can form a wide, valveless conduit directly from the pelvis or extremity to the central veins. Thrombosis in these veins carries a high risk of pulmonary embolism, which is a well-recognised cause of sudden death in young adults with this disease (4).

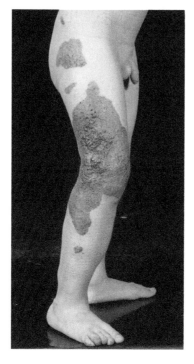

FIGURE 12.1 Image of a 4-year-old boy with Klippel–Trénaunay syndrome (KTS) affecting his right lower limb.

## ABERRANT MUSCLE SYNDROME

Typically, this is characterised by unilateral muscular hyperplasia, aberrant muscles or accessory muscles, ulnar drift of the fingers in the metacarpophalangeal (MP) joints, flexion contractures of the MP joints, extension contractures of the wrist, and enlargement of the spaces between the metacarpals. This can also present with segmental muscle overgrowth of the foot and ankle. Aberrant muscle syndrome tends not to present with specific vascular malformations.

## FIBROADIPOSE VASCULAR ANOMALY (FAVA)

FAVA is an unusual vascular anomaly that is often initially misdiagnosed as a venous malformation. Patients typically present at primary school age with progressive, severe pain which is typically disproportionate to the clinical or imaging findings. The calf (typically the gastrocnemius and/or soleus muscles) and the forearm muscles are most commonly affected, but FAVA can occur in subcutaneous fat or other tissue types. It is characterised by dense infiltrative tissue that typically involves individual muscle groups and encases neurovascular structures (5–7) (Figure 12.2). It is often, but not always, associated with large calibre dysplastic veins (phlebectasia) running through the lesion. MRI imaging can be misleading, as the lesions appear similar to venous malformations; the diagnostic key is found on ultrasound imaging, which demonstrates highly echogenic tissue which casts a dense acoustic shadow (Figure 12.3). This is very different to the ultrasound features of a venous malformation. Although FAVA has rather bland histological features, biopsy may be useful in excluding other diagnoses. In many cases, FAVA is a diagnosis of exclusion.

Some lesions remain small and relatively insignificant, but a large proportion of lesions display a progressive growth pattern over time, crossing fascial planes and invading adjacent muscle compartments. Progressive muscle contractures, resulting in loss of joint range of motion and intractable, debilitating pain are often seen in patients with advanced disease. Patients with a diagnosis of FAVA require an individualised treatment approach, including physiotherapy and pain management. Sclerotherapy of the dysplastic veins is rarely helpful in terms of symptom control but may be helpful prior to more definitive intervention, such as cryoablation or surgical debulking, which is discussed in more detail below (4). The challenge is knowing when to intervene, as some lesions are relentlessly progressive over time and others are not.

## RASA1 AND EPHB4-REGULATED DISORDERS

Germline loss-of-function mutations in *RASA1* and *EPHB4* give rise to capillary malformation-arteriovenous malformation (CM-AVM) syndrome Types 1 and 2, respectively (8, 9). These hereditary vascular syndromes have high penetrance and variable expressivity with considerable phenotypic diversity even within families. These germline heterozygous mutations predispose to development of a number of vascular anomalies with a second somatic hit (genetic variant) in the affected lesion (8–10). CM-AVM 1 and 2 are characterised by classic cutaneous lesions: multifocal, pink-to-red cutaneous capillary stains on the face, body, and limbs. These can range in size from <1 cm to >15 cm and are often observed with a surrounding pale halo. They can be warm to the touch and are thought by some to represent small micro-arteriovenous fistulas (AVFs) rather than true capillary malformations. In addition, in CM-AVM 2, telangiectasia can be observed, most commonly on the lips and face. Affected individuals may have an associated AVM or AVF which may be cerebral, spinal, subcutaneous, intra-muscular, or bony and are reported in over

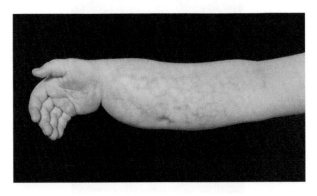

FIGURE 12.2 Image of a teenage boy with FAVA affecting his right forearm. The surgical scar is from previous debulking surgery. Note the contracture at the wrist.

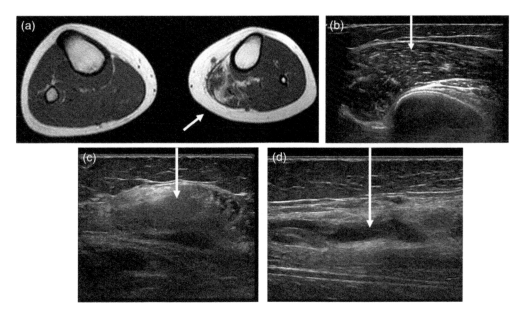

FIGURE 12.3 Imaging in a child with a FAVA lesion of the left calf, demonstrating (a) patchy, non-descript signal change and volume loss in the medial gastrocnemius (arrow) and wasting of all the left calf muscles compared to the right; (b) normal ultrasound appearances of the quadriceps muscle (arrow); (c) in contrast, the left calf muscles appear markedly echogenic (arrow) and cast an acoustic shadow; (d) a few dysplastic venous channels run through the centre of the lesion.

one-third of cases. Parkes Weber syndrome describes a cutaneous vascular skin stain secondary to multiple micro-AVFs affecting a limb with associated soft tissue and skeletal hypertrophy, typically resulting in a limb length discrepancy (Figure 12.4). Germline variants are inherited in an autosomal dominant manner with a 50% chance of passing on the genetic change to offspring. Affected families should be referred to a clinical genetics team to facilitate genetic screening and counselling of family members.

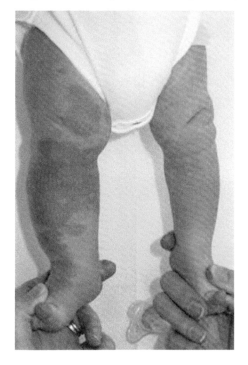

FIGURE 12.4 Image of an infant with Parkes Weber syndrome of the right leg, with a cutaneous vascular skin stain secondary to multiple micro-AVFs throughout the limb and associated soft tissue and skeletal hypertrophy.

## *PTEN*-RELATED DISORDERS

Heterozygous germline mutations in the tumour suppressor gene phosphatase and tensin homolog (*PTEN*) result in PTEN hamartoma syndrome (PTEN-HS), a cancer predisposition syndrome characterised by the development of multiple hamartomas in different tissues. *PTEN* is a negative regulator of *PIK3CA*; therefore, mutations in *PTEN* result in activation of the PI3K-AKT-mTOR pathway. PTEN-HS describes a spectrum of disorders and includes the clinically delineated syndromes: Cowden syndrome, Bannayan–Riley–Ruvalcaba syndrome, multiple hamartoma syndrome, and *PTEN*-related Proteus syndrome. PTEN-HS can present with developmental delay, macrocephaly, penile freckling, and social communication disorders. PTEN-HS patients have an increased risk of benign and also malignant tumour development, most commonly of the breast, thyroid, and endometrium, and require appropriate surveillance in late childhood and throughout adulthood.

PTEN hamartoma of soft tissue (PHOST) describes an intra-muscular fast-flow vascular anomaly observed in PTEN-HS (11). Clinically, PHOST lesions present with pain and swelling, often with overlying vascular discolouration of the skin, most commonly affecting the lower limbs, followed by the upper limbs, trunk, head, and neck (Figure 12.5). Similar to other high-flow lesions, such as sporadic AVMs, high-output cardiac failure has rarely been described in the advanced stages of the disease. Histologically, PHOST shows vascular components with vascular clusters and large draining veins and a variable amount of fat and fibrous tissue. Although lesions are predominantly intra-muscular, the fascia, subcutis, and dermis are frequently involved.

Imaging features in this condition are very hetereogeneous, often show a poorly demarcated, often multifocal intra-muscular high-flow vascular lesion with a variable fatty component. Angiography can demonstrate multiple AVFs.

PHOST can be difficult to differentiate clinically and histologically from sporadic vascular anomalies such as FAVA and AVMs. Often vascular anomalies in *PTEN* follow an aggressive course with rapid recurrence despite intervention. This highlights the need for a full systems examination, including head circumference, in all children presenting with vascular anomalies, as early identification of syndromes such as PTEN-HS will enable appropriate developmental support and tumour surveillance as well as genetic screening of potentially affected family members.

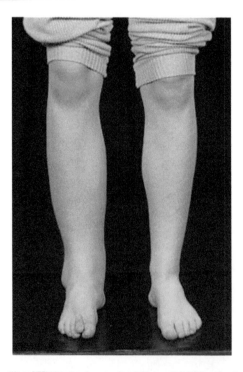

FIGURE 12.5 Image of a child with a PTEN hamartoma of soft tissue (PHOST) affecting the right lower limb.

## PROTEUS SYNDROME

Proteus syndrome is a mosaic overgrowth syndrome characterised by progressive, asymmetric dysregulated overgrowth of various tissues. Clinical manifestations include skeletal overgrowth, epidermal and connective tissue naevi, vascular anomalies, and adipocyte overgrowth. Pathognomonic cerebriform connective tissue naevi are present in some patients but are not required for diagnosis. In comparison to PROS, the overgrowth in Proteus syndrome is progressive and disproportionate. Extensive slow-flow vascular malformations can predispose to venous thromboembolism. Venous thrombosis leading to pulmonary thromboembolism is a recognised cause of sudden death in young adults. There is an increased risk of tumour development, most frequently benign tumours of the ovary or salivary gland, or meningiomas. Proteus is caused by a recurrent somatic activating mutation in the gene *AKT1* (12). Early genotyping of children presenting with segmental overgrowth syndromes is critical to identify the rare subtype of Proteus syndrome, which follows an aggressive postnatal course and is more likely to require early intervention and treatment.

## *PIK3R1*-RELATED OVERGROWTH SPECTRUM

Somatic activating mutations in the gene *PIK3R1* have recently been identified as a cause of segmental overgrowth and vascular anomalies in clinical phenotypes clinically indistinguishable from PROS (13). *PIK3R1* encodes the p85α, p55α, and p50α regulatory subunits of PI3K, and activating mutation results in overactivation of the PI3K-AKT-mTOR pathway. Clinically, patients present with mixed vascular anomalies, a wide sandal gap, macrodactyly, lymphatic malformations, and overgrowth of soft tissue and bone. Although this appears to be a much rarer genetic cause of this clinical spectrum than mutations in *PIK3CA*, genetic testing for mutations in *PIK3R1* from the affected tissue of patients who present with compatible features but who are found to be *PIK3CA* mutation negative will be important in appropriately stratifying patients for future targeted medical therapies.

## CLINICAL ASSESSMENT

All children require a comprehensive clinical examination. The clinical assessment focuses on the following features:

- Features related to the overgrowth/complex vascular anomaly
- Cutaneous features
- Acral limb malformations
- Skeletal assessment
- Neurological assessment
- Surveillance for associated tumours

Assessment of the extent of the overgrowth and/or complex vascular anomaly is performed noting site, size, shape, depth, and consistency. The overgrowth or complex vascular anomaly may affect the upper or lower limbs and, in more complex syndromes, both upper and lower limbs with asymmetrical truncal involvement. Hemifacial hypertrophy may occur in CLOVES and PTEN-HS, and a complete cranial nerve examination should be performed.

A thorough cutaneous examination noting any skin changes such as epidermal naevi and vascular malformations is extremely important and can help guide diagnosis. It is important to include assessment of any mucosal changes peri- and intra-orally, peri-anally, and on the perineum, looking for papillomatous lesions and venous malformations.

Complex vascular anomalies and segmental overgrowth pathologies such as FAVA and aberrant muscle syndrome require full assessment of upper and lower limbs, noting problems with active and passive range of motion. It is imperative to perform a full neurovascular assessment of the upper and lower limbs as compressive neuropathies can be a complicating sequalae of some segmental overgrowth syndromes. Hand therapy and physiotherapy involvement is extremely important in obtaining baseline assessments of key upper and lower limb functions.

Scoliosis, recurrent patellar subluxation, rarely bilateral genu recurvatum, and hyperextensible joints are potential sequelae of overgrowth syndromes and complex vascular anomalies. Orthopaedic assessment is extremely important to rule out these issues, monitor their progression, and treat accordingly.

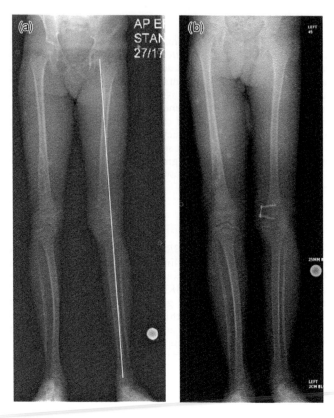

FIGURE 12.6 Serial standing leg length and alignment radiographs of a skeletally immature child with a complex vascular anomaly affecting both lower limbs. (a) The white line passes lateral to the middle half of the left knee, indicating a valgus deformity and increased loading of her arthritic medial compartment of the knee. (b) Following guided growth, the mechanical alignment has improved, as have her knee symptoms.

Leg-length discrepancies are measured by leg-length measurement assessments, gait analysis, and imaging (Figure 12.6).

The central nervous system can be affected; a history of seizures and developmental delay requires review and assessment by a paediatric neurologist. It is extremely important to assess for macrocephaly with regular head circumference measurements. This is commonly seen in MCAP and PTEN-HS. Assessment for posterior spina bifida is important in fibroadipose overgrowth syndrome (FAO).

## IMAGING

Plain radiographs can be used to assess osseous changes such as overgrowth, deformities, flexion contractures, arthropathy, osteopenia, and leg-length discrepancy. They may also be key in excluding an unsuspected skeletal dysplasia.

Ultrasonography (US) is a dynamic evaluation tool that provides real-time imaging of the vascular anatomy and pathology (e.g., venous ectasia and incompetence, flow stagnation, and venous thrombosis) as well as vascular malformations. US is useful for initial assessment of painful episodes in patients with complex vascular anomalies and overgrowth syndromes. It may differentiate between thrombophlebitis and lymphangitis. US is very useful for assessing blood flow within malformations and guiding the judicious application of angiographic cross-sectional imaging such as computed tomography (CT) angiography and magnetic resonance (MR) angiography or venography, which can be time consuming and is often over-requested.

In selected cases, direct fluoroscopic venography has value in mapping complex venous anatomy, particularly for persistent marginal veins, when the pattern of venous drainage has important management implications (Figure 12.7).

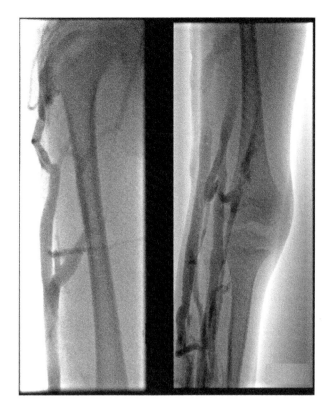

FIGURE 12.7 Fluoroscopic images of a venogram of the right lower limb of a teenager with a complex marginal vein, showing multiple lateral marginal veins below the knee, some of which drain into a deep system (which is not fully opacified yet on these images) just above the knee. A single marginal vein persists in the thigh, splitting into numerous smaller veins as it courses through the gluteal muscles and into the deep pelvic veins.

CT is often key to delineating complex osseous changes. Three-dimensional (3D) image reconstruction can be valuable for surgical planning. MRI is immensely valuable in assessing soft tissue involvement and the composition of any vascular anomaly and overgrowth. It can also reveal unsuspected components such as a persistent marginal venous system in the affected limb.

## BIOPSY AND OTHER INVESTIGATIONS

Commonly, a biopsy is required to define the exact pathology of the vascular anomaly or overgrowth. In addition, for somatic overgrowth syndromes secondary to *PIK3CA* and *AKT1*, DNA extracted directly from affected tissue is key to obtaining a genetic diagnosis which may be used to inform prognosis and guide medical management. For superficial lesions in patients without a significant bleeding risk, this can be performed under local anaesthetic via a simple punch biopsy. For deep lesions or lesions in patients with a coagulopathy, biopsies should be performed by an interventional radiologist or a surgeon, and when necessary, there should be peri-procedural input from a haematologist experienced in this field. Histopathology can help differentiate between conditions with clinical overlap such as FAVA and PHOST. In mosaic syndromes, DNA extracted directly from affected tissue is necessary to establish genotype, which can help with diagnosis, inform prognosis, and direct patients to the appropriate targeted medical therapy. For germline conditions such as CM-AVM syndrome and PTEN-HS, leucocyte DNA extracted from blood can be used for genetic testing of relevant genes.

## HISTOPATHOLOGY

The histological features of many of these conditions are often non-specific and clinical context is key.

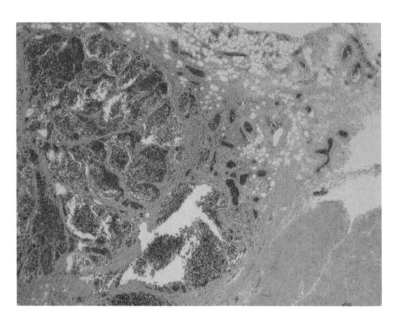

FIGURE 12.8 Photomicrograph of FAVA, H&E staining, demonstrating fibrous tissue, fat, and muscle admixed with a poorly circumscribed vascular anomaly comprising irregularly shaped thin-walled vascular channels, many of which contain blood, representing a mixture of venous and lymphatic type vascular channels (original magnification x40).

## MEDICAL MANAGEMENT

Advances in our understanding of the genetic basis of many complex vascular anomalies and overgrowth syndromes has enabled the use of several targeted medical therapies for these cohorts.

Sirolimus is a mammalian target of rapamycin (mTOR) inhibitor. mTOR is a serine/threonine-specific protein kinase which lies downstream of PI3K and AKT in the PI3K-AKT-mTOR growth signalling pathway. Sirolimus can be an effective medical therapy in PROS, with evidence suggesting it can modestly reduce overgrowth and improve pain and mobility (14). Sirolimus has also been used in PTEN-HS vascular anomalies leading to reduction in size and associated pain in some high-flow vascular anomalies (15–17).

Alpelisib is a specific inhibitor of p110α and, therefore, a more directly targeted therapy for somatic mutations in *PIK3CA*. Recently, it has been demonstrated to be safe and effective in a compassionate-use series of 19 adults with *PIK3CA*-related overgrowth syndrome, leading to an improvement in clinical symptoms in all patients, including reduced fatigue, decrease in size of vascular anomalies, improvement in scoliosis, reduction in weight, and an improvement in cerebral perfusion in two patients with MCAPs (18). The side effect profile in this cohort was favourable.

The MEK inhibitor trametinib has been shown to improve AVM-associated cardiac failure in a single case of CM-AVM 2 (19). As with sporadic AVMs, MEK inhibition may be an effective treatment for CM-AVM associated AVMs in symptomatic patients whose lesions are not amenable to surgery or embolisation.

Pan-AKT inhibitors, such as miransertib, have shown safety and efficacy in patients with Proteus syndrome in small case series and reports, with slowing of the progression of overgrowth and improvements in pain and quality of life (20).

## LASER MANAGEMENT

For superficial elements of complex vascular anomalies and overgrowth, laser treatment can be very effective. Cutaneous capillary and lymphatic malformations may be treated with laser therapy if they bleed or are crusted. There are two types of lasers available: pulsed dye laser is effective in lightening capillary malformations, whereas ablative $CO_2$ lasers are used to control leakage and bleeding from lymphatic vesicles.

## INTERVENTIONAL RADIOLOGY MANAGEMENT

Interventional radiology (IR) can bring value to the work-up and management of selected patients in this markedly diverse cohort. Catheter angiography remains the gold standard for vascular mapping of high-flow lesions, and in children, direct venography is usually performed by an interventional radiologist. Such vascular imaging is often helpful in multidisciplinary discussions regarding surgical or endovascular management options. Embolisation of high-flow lesions has value as the definitive treatment in some cases or can be used pre-operatively in surgical candidates to reduce the vascularity of the surgical field and decrease intra-operative blood loss.

Sclerotherapy is often an attractive option for low-flow components of a malformation, as discussed in Chapters 8 and 10, again, either as a definitive treatment or with the aim of downsizing the lesion prior to surgical debulking. Doxycycline sclerotherapy of postsurgical seroma cavities is sometimes offered and can be useful in reducing postoperative recovery times.

Increasingly, IR contributes more innovative procedures to the multi-disciplinary management of these patients. Interventions include cryoablation for selected FAVA lesions (21) and other solid malformations, and endovenous laser ablation (EVLT) and/or embolisation of large dysplastic veins, such as persistent marginal veins. Closure of these veins in childhood is important, both because they become a major cause of limb swelling and pain in later life when they are then too large to be easily managed surgically and because they are a source of potentially fatal thromboembolism (4, 22). For this second reason, it is important not only to close the vein with endovenous laser and/or sclerotherapy but also to embolise the top of the vein before the point that it drains into the central veins to prevent postintervention thrombus from travelling centrally.

## SURGICAL MANAGEMENT

Surgical management is tailored toward managing patients' symptoms and functional deficits and maintaining their quality of life (QoL). If timed correctly, surgery may also be preventative; it may limit or reverse progressive change in limb length or alignment, for example. Surgical intervention may vary from simple excision or debulking surgery, through tendon rebalancing procedures and correction of bone and joint deformity, to, in some cases, amputation (Figure 12.9).

The aims of the surgery vary depending on the clinical picture, the patient, and the family. It is essential that a holistic approach is employed and that the family and the patient understand what the outcomes are likely to be.

Typically, the surgical procedures fit into one of the following categories:

- Simple excision or debulking or soft tissues and/or bone.
- Release of contractures and/or prevention of joint subluxation.
- Tendon rebalancing procedures.
- Amputation, from limited procedures for overgrown digits or rays to more extensive procedures, such as through knee amputation.
- Management of limb length discrepancies and/or management of the length (but not so easily the bulk) of toes and fingers.
    a. Treatments include those that manipulate or guide the growth, such as temporary or permanent epiphysiodesis.
    b. Osteotomies may also be used to correct deformity.
- Joint fusion (arthrodesis) may also play a role.
- Surface coblative treatments.

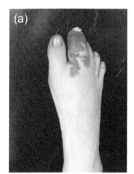
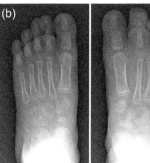
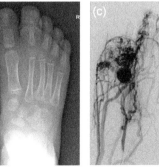
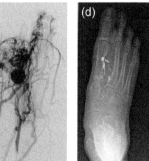

FIGURE 12.9 Images of the right foot of a 6-year-old girl with a high-flow malformation affecting the right second ray. The (a) photograph and (b) plain radiograph demonstrate overgrowth and of the second ray; (c) an angiogram image demonstrates the nidus of the malformation. This was treated by pre-surgical embolisation and then ray excision. (d) The final radiograph was taken after the second ray amputation, with high-density (white) embolic material in the residual embolised vessels of the arteriovenous malformation.

There are multiple situations in which surgical intervention should be considered, but once the significant risks of surgery have been balanced against the realistic benefits of such intervention, there are fewer situations in which surgery is actually performed. Patients suffering with severe pain, neurological deficit due to compression, functional deficits due to joint contracture and large vascular anomalies, and overgrowth syndromes causing abnormal resting postures may all be candidates for a surgical procedure, particularly if other options such as IR treatments are not practical (Figure 12.10). Surgery to improve quality of life (QoL) is an individual decision between the family, the multi-disciplinary team, and the surgeon and may be indicated to improve cosmesis, facilitate shoe wear, and improve mobility and independence.

Pre-operative planning is extremely important and the key to successful surgery. Some patients with complex vascular anomalies and overgrowth have a higher risk of coagulopathy and thromboembolism; involvement of a haematologist with experience in this field is essential regarding anticoagulation regimes required pre-operatively, peri-operatively, and postoperatively. Massive transfusion protocols may be required for large debulking procedures. Complications are related to the two linked potential risks of bleeding and thrombosis. Please refer to Chapter 3 for further details.

Complex vascular anomalies and overgrowth syndromes can present with intractable pain and joint contracture (Figure 12.11). They may also present with neurological deficits due to nerve compression. Debulking aims to reduce symptoms and improve functional deficits. Occasionally, excisional surgery aims to improve limb range of motion and position. For large vascular malformations involving the limbs, debulking can help reduce the circumference of the limb to improve the patient's resting functional position and cosmesis.

*PIK3CA*-related overgrowth disorders such as aberrant muscle syndrome (AMS) and FAVA can present with functional deficits due to contracture of the involved muscle-tendon unit.

In FAVA particularly, the pain from the lesion is associated with a reluctance for the child to move (i.e., stretch) the muscle and, hence, the joint, leading to secondary contractures. Typically, AMS presents with hypertrophied intrinsic muscles resulting in the hand resting in an intrinsic plus position (Figure 12.12). Commonly, this requires debulking of the lumbrical muscles and splinting and stretching to improve tendon imbalance.

One of the main indications for surgical management in patients with FAVA is pain with a secondary joint contracture. Once the lesion has been excised, the contracture can be addressed by a variety of techniques that include lengthening of the muscle-tendon unit, release of joint contractures, and/or

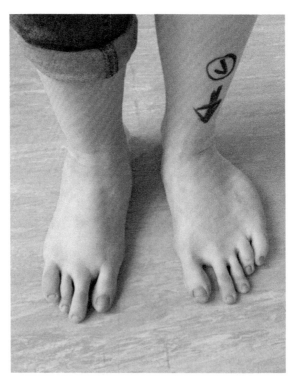

FIGURE 12.10 Teenage girl with *PIK3CA*-related overgrowth spectrum (PROS) who underwent surgery for a right second ray amputation for overgrowth. She was pleased with the result and awaits surgery on her left side.

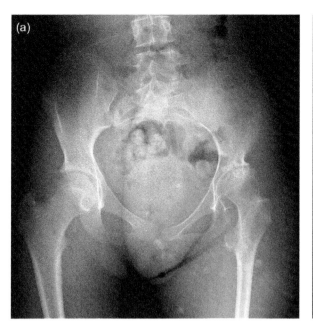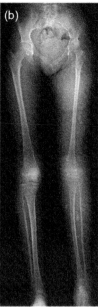

FIGURE 12.11 Pelvis radiograph of a teenage girl with a venous malformation of the left leg, highlighting (a) marked degenerative change (arthritis) in the left hip joint secondary to multiple intra-articular bleeds; (b) the long leg radiograph demonstrates multiple phleboliths in the soft tissues and an apparent shortening of the left leg due to her flexed knee and hip position secondary to the pain and stiffness in her joints.

osteotomy to ensure the joint and limb position is improved and a satisfactory passive range of movement is obtained. Maintenance of this improved range may require use of a splint such as an ankle foot orthosis (AFO) and/or a tendon transfer procedure. The child will not regain normal function due to excision of the muscle mass which contains the FAVA, but the relief of pain secondary to excision does encourage a more normal use of the limb and, hence, overall function is improved by excision of the lesion.

Infrequently, surgical amputation is required to manage intractable pain and immobility, contractures, and/or simply a very bulky/heavy limb which has little useful function. This particular surgical treatment should not be undertaken lightly and requires extensive, repeated discussion with the patient and family with early involvement with a prosthetist familiar with the particular needs of this patient group. It is important to understand that the use of a prosthetic limb following such an amputation is

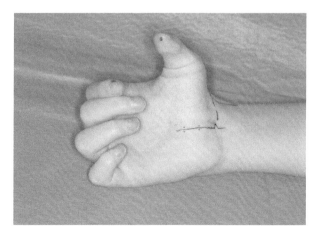

FIGURE 12.12 Pre-operative image of the right hand of a girl with aberrant muscle syndrome (AMS) affecting the thenar eminence.

unusually difficult, as the remaining limb is frequently also affected by the vascular/overgrowth abnormality, and getting an artificial limb to 'fit' comfortably and to be useful is uncommon.

In some infants with a large vascular malformation and associated high-output cardiac failure, amputation can be lifesaving. In other circumstances, it can be life-enhancing. Whilst mobility might be improved, it rarely allows walking with a prosthetic limb. A ray amputation of the foot or hand improves bulk, appearance, and function and may allow improved use of shoe wear.

Controlled ablation (coblation), a bipolar plasma device designed to operate at a relatively low temperature, dissolves a particular type of tissue. It causes minimal damage to surrounding healthy tissue and coagulates blood vessels. In certain cases of superficial, localised microcystic lymphatic and venous malformations, such as those involving skin or mucosal surfaces, coblation can be a useful surgical tool in managing symptoms such as bleeding.

Surgical debulking procedures result in scar formation and early engagement with the physiotherapist, hand therapist, and occupational therapist is important to implement scar management strategies and maintain joint and muscle function.

The postoperative follow-up required by patients with complex vascular anomalies and overgrowth is varied and depends on the surgical treatment performed. Healing wounds are monitored for infection, wound dehiscence, and haematoma. All debulking, tendon rebalancing surgeries, and amputations require wound reviews to make sure complete healing occurs. This can be performed on an outpatient basis. Any hand or foot surgery requires early input from hand therapists and physiotherapists. Customised splints may be required for specific tendon rebalancing procedures of the hand and foot. Guided postoperative hand and foot exercises with the therapist are extremely important after tendon rebalancing procedures to optimise subsequent range of motion.

As the child grows, there may be an increasing discrepancy between the length and alignment of the limbs. This is most noticeable in the lower limbs and may limit function and quality of life. If a limb length discrepancy is predicted to be more than 2–2.5 cm at skeletal maturity, then an epiphysiodesis of either the distal femoral or proximal tibial (or both) physis is undertaken at an appropriate age (usually between ages 10–14). Similarly, if the mechanical alignment of the limb demonstrates progressive change, then surgical intervention to guide the growth for a period of time may prevent progression and/or achieve correction of limb alignment. Both epiphysiodesis and guided growth techniques are small interventions with few significant risks (23).

Joint subluxation and dislocations do occur and are difficult to treat due to the vascularity of the surrounding soft tissues. The overall function of such a limb is often poor due to the extensive abnormality and the added effect of a joint subluxation may be relatively small. In such cases, the risks of surgery seem relatively higher.

There are a number of key ongoing issues that must be monitored as symptoms of aches and pains and development of contractures worsens during growth spells and become problematic. The conditions can worsen during hormonal changes such as puberty. Follow-up is critical, as there is a high degree of neuropathic pain and rebound pain.

---

## KEY MESSAGES

- Complex vascular anomalies and overgrowth syndromes are a spectrum of multi-system conditions which require a multidisciplinary approach to management.

- Routine genetic testing of this cohort is recommended to inform prognosis, determine eligibility for medical therapy, and enable genetic counselling and screening of potentially affected family members in the case of hereditary germline syndromes.

- Many of these conditions confer an increased risk of thromboembolism, and those at risk require input from a paediatric haematologist.

- Multiple imaging modalities may be required, as these complex syndromes often affect multiple tissue types.

- Many children will require surgical input from a specialist team, which may include orthopaedics, plastic surgery, urology, general surgery, maxillofacial surgery, and interventional radiology as well as input from physiotherapy, occupational therapy, and orthotics services.

# REFERENCES

1. Keppler-Noreuil, K.M., Rios, J.J., Parker, V.E., Semple, R.K., Lindhurst, M.J., Sapp, J.C., Alomari, A., Ezaki, M., Dobyns, W., and Biesecker, L.G. (2015). PIK3CA-related overgrowth spectrum (PROS): Diagnostic and testing eligibility criteria, differential diagnosis, and evaluation. *Am J Med Genet A* 167A, 287–295.
2. Hol, J.A., Jewell, R., Chowdhury, T., Duncan, C., Nakata, K., Oue, T., Gauthier-Villars, M., Littooij, A.S., Kaneko, Y., Graf, N., et al. (2021). Wilms tumour surveillance in at-risk children: Literature review and recommendations from the SIOP-Europe Host Genome Working Group and SIOP renal tumour study group. *Eur J Cancer* 153, 51–63.
3. Harnarayan, P., and Harnanan, D. (2022). The Klippel-Trénaunay syndrome in 2022: Unravelling its genetic and molecular profile and its link to the limb overgrowth syndromes. *Vasc Health Risk Manag* 18, 201–209.
4. Reis, J., 3rd, Alomari, A.I., Trenor, C.C., 3rd, Adams, D.M., Fishman, S.J., Spencer, S.A., Shaikh, R., Lillis, A.P., Surnedi, M.K., and Chaudry, G. (2018). Pulmonary thromboembolic events in patients with congenital lipomatous overgrowth, vascular malformations, epidermal nevi, and spinal/skeletal abnormalities and Klippel-Trénaunay syndrome. *J Vasc Surg Venous Lymphat Disord* 6, 511–516.
5. Alomari, A.K., Glusac, E.J., Choi, J., Hui, P., Seeley, E.H., Caprioli, R.M., Watsky, K.L., Urban, J., and Lazova, R. (2015). Congenital nevi versus metastatic melanoma in a newborn to a mother with malignant melanoma – Diagnosis supported by sex chromosome analysis and imaging mass spectrometry. *Journal of Cutaneous Pathology* 42(10), 757–764. doi: 10.1111/cup.12523 PMID: 25989266.
6. Lipede, C., Nikkhah, D., Ashton, R., Murphy, G., Barnacle, A.M., Patel, P.A., Smith, G.D., Eastwood, D.M., and Sivakumar, B. (2021). Management of fibro-adipose vascular anomalies (FAVA) in paediatric practice. *Jpras Open* 29, 71–81.
7. Cheung, K., Taghinia, A.H., Sood, R.F., Alomari, A.I., Spencer, S.A., Al-Ibraheemi, A., Kozakewich, H.P.W., Chaudry, G., Greene, A.K., Mulliken, J.B., et al. (2020). Fibroadipose vascular anomaly in the upper extremity: A distinct entity with characteristic clinical, radiological, and histopathological findings. *J Hand Surg Am* 45, 68.e61–68.e13.
8. Eerola, I., Boon, L.M., Mulliken, J.B., Burrows, P.E., Dompmartin, A., Watanabe, S., Vanwijck, R., and Vikkula, M. (2003). Capillary malformation-arteriovenous malformation, a new clinical and genetic disorder caused by RASA1 mutations. *Am J Hum Genet* 73, 1240–1249.
9. Amyere, M., Revencu, N., Helaers, R., Pairet, E., Baselga, E., Cordisco, M., Chung, W., Dubois, J., Lacour, J.P., Martorell, L., et al. (2017). Germline loss-of-function mutations in EPHB4 cause a second form of capillary malformation-arteriovenous malformation (CM-AVM2) deregulating RAS-MAPK signaling. *Circulation* 136, 1037–1048.
10. Lapinski, P.E., Doosti, A., Salato, V., North, P., Burrows, P.E., and King, P.D. (2018). Somatic second hit mutation of RASA1 in vascular endothelial cells in capillary-malformation-arteriovenous malformation. *Eur J Med Genet* 61, 11–16.
11. Kurek, K.C., Howard, E., Tennant, L.B., Upton, J., Alomari, A.I., Burrows, P.E., Chalache, K., Harris, D.J., Trenor, C.C., 3rd, Eng, C., et al. (2012). PTEN hamartoma of soft tissue: A distinctive lesion in PTEN syndromes. *Am J Surg Pathol* 36, 671–687.
12. Lindhurst, M.J., Sapp, J.C., Teer, J.K., Johnston, J.J., Finn, E.M., Peters, K., Turner, J., Cannons, J.L., Bick, D., Blakemore, L., et al. (2011). A mosaic activating mutation in AKT1 associated with the Proteus syndrome. *N Engl J Med* 365, 611–619.
13. Cottrell, C.E., Bender, N.R., Zimmermann, M.T., Heusel, J.W., Corliss, M., Evenson, M.J., Magrini, V., Corsmeier, D.J., Avenarius, M., Dudley, J.N., et al. (2021). Somatic PIK3R1 variation as a cause of vascular malformations and overgrowth. *Genet Med: Off J Am Col Med Genet* 23, 1882–1888.
14. Parker, V.E.R., Keppler-Noreuil, K.M., Faivre, L., Luu, M., Oden, N.L., De Silva, L., Sapp, J.C., Andrews, K., Bardou, M., Chen, K.Y., et al. (2019). Safety and efficacy of low-dose sirolimus in the *PIK3CA*-related overgrowth spectrum. *Genet Med: Off J Am Col Med Genet* 21, 1189–1198.
15. Liu, L.Y., Jeng, M.R., and Teng, J.M.C. (2022). Inhibiting PI3K and MAPK pathways: Clinical response in PTEN syndrome. *Journal of Vascular Anomalies* 3, e047.
16. Komiya, T., Blumenthal, G.M., DeChowdhury, R., Fioravanti, S., Ballas, M.S., Morris, J., Hornyak, T.J., Wank, S., Hewitt, S.M., Morrow, B., et al. (2019). A pilot study of sirolimus in subjects with cowden syndrome or other syndromes characterized by germline mutations in PTEN. *Oncologist* 24, 1510-e1265.
17. Adams, D.M., Trenor, C.C., 3rd, Hammill, A.M., Vinks, A.A., Patel, M.N., Chaudry, G., Wentzel, M.S., Mobberley-Schuman, P.S., Campbell, L.M., Brookbank, C., et al. (2016). Efficacy and safety of sirolimus in the treatment of complicated vascular anomalies. *Pediatrics* 137, e20153257.
18. Delestre, F., Venot, Q., Bayard, C., Fraissenon, A., Ladraa, S., Hoguin, C., Chapelle, C., Yamaguchi, J., Cassaca, R., Zerbib, L., et al. (2021). Alpelisib administration reduced lymphatic malformations in a mouse model and in patients. *Sci Transl Med* 13, eabg0809.
19. Nicholson, C.L., Flanagan, S., Murati, M., Boull, C., McGough, E., Ameduri, R., Weigel, B., and Maguiness, S. (2022). Successful management of an arteriovenous malformation with trametinib in a patient with capillary-malformation arteriovenous malformation syndrome and cardiac compromise. *Pediatr Dermatol* 39(2), 316–319. doi: 10.1111/pde.14912.
20. Ours, C.A., Sapp, J.C., Hodges, M.B., de Moya, A.J., and Biesecker, L.G. (2021). Case report: Five-year experience of AKT inhibition with miransertib (MK-7075) in an individual with proteus syndrome. *Cold Spring Harb Mol Case Stud* 7(6), a006134. doi: 10.1101/mcs.a006134.
21. Shaikh, R., Alomari, A.I., Kerr, C.L., Miller, P., and Spencer, S.A. (2016). Cryoablation in fibro-adipose vascular anomaly (FAVA): A minimally invasive treatment option. *Pediatr Radiol* 46, 1179–1186.
22. King, K., Landrigan-Ossar, M., Clemens, R., Chaudry, G., and Alomari, A.I. (2013). The use of endovenous laser treatment in toddlers. *J Vasc Interv Radiol* 24, 855–858.
23. Memarzadeh, A., Pengas, I., Syed, S., and Eastwood, D.M. (2014). Limb length discrepancy in cutis marmorata telangiectatica congenita: An audit of assessment and management in a multidisciplinary setting. *Br J Dermatol* 170, 681–686.

# Orbital Vascular Malformations

**13**

Sri Gore, Alex Barnacle, and Fergus Robertson

## INTRODUCTION

All vascular anomaly types can occur in the orbit. Infantile haemangiomas are common and can affect the orbit and peri-orbital soft tissues, but other vascular anomalies of the orbit are rare. Other diagnoses such as transcranial shunts (caroticocavernous fistulas), which are predominantly seen in adults, and orbital tumours must be considered. These cases are best managed by an experienced multidisciplinary team comprising an oculoplastic surgeon, orthoptist, and interventional radiologist.

The most common scenario encountered with regard to haemangiomas in or around the orbit is obstruction or malpositioning of an infant's visual axis, which threatens the normal development of their visual pathways. This situation must be recognised early and the baby referred on to a specialist team for urgent assessment and further management. As detailed in Chapter 5, the medical treatment of infantile haemangiomas is straightforward and effective, but treatment must be started early, during the proliferative phase of growth.

Vascular malformations of the orbit are rare. Low-flow malformations present more frequently in children than high-flow lesions, though this incidence ratio is usually reversed in adults (1). In the authors' experience, lymphatic malformations (LMs) are seen far more commonly than venous malformations (VMs) in the orbit, though other centres report differing experiences (1).

The clinical presentation and the principles of management of the spectrum of vascular malformations are broadly the same in the orbit as they are elsewhere in the body and are fully discussed elsewhere in this book. This chapter will focus on some key differences in presentation, natural history, and management of these lesions when they affect the orbit or peri-orbital soft tissues (2).

## CLINICAL PRESENTATION

### LYMPHATIC MALFORMATIONS

LMs of the orbit tend to present in one of two ways. They are not usually apparent at birth. They can present at any age but are seen more commonly in childhood. The cysts may slowly increase in size over weeks or months, presenting with asymmetry of the orbits as the mass effect becomes more obvious (Figure 13.1). Those that present acutely have usually been undetectable and asymptomatic until a spontaneous bleed into the cysts causes sudden expansion of the malformation. If the cysts are in the posterior orbit, this causes sudden and often dramatic proptosis, which can be exceptionally painful. The resultant stretching of the optic nerve and raised intra-orbital pressure often affects visual function, and visual acuity can drop significantly. If the cysts are extra-conal or pre-septal, the peri-orbital soft tissues can appear swollen and the eye closed. If the lymphatic tissue involves the medial canthus, the caruncle itself can be enlarged and discoloured. Because the lymphatic tissue in a malformation responds to even mild systemic inflammatory symptoms by producing fluid, there is often a history of fluctuating swelling and discomfort directly related to patterns of systemic illness such as a viral upper respiratory tract infection.

Lymphatic involvement of the peri-ocular tissues can present as thickening of lids, bulkiness of the medial caruncle, or thickening of the sclera or caruncle (Figure 13.1). Note that lymphatic involvement

146

DOI: 10.1201/9781003257417-13

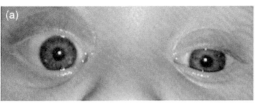
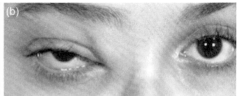

FIGURE 13.1 (a) Progressive right sided proptosis in a 6-month-old child secondary to an enlarging posterior orbital lymphatic malformation. (b) The typical appearance of lymphatic involvement of the pre-septal soft tissues of the right orbit in a 7-year-old child.

of the skin itself or the caruncle can be deep red or purple in colour, and any bleed into subcutaneous cysts can give a purple 'bruised' hue to the skin. This is often misinterpreted as suggesting the malformation is venous in origin.

## VENOUS MALFORMATIONS

VMs of the orbit typically have a more subtle presentation. They usually behave like small venous varices, increasing in size with Valsalva manoeuvres and changes in body position. So, they may be more symptomatic with sports such as gymnastics, when reading or writing for long periods with the head tilted down, or with everyday activities such as tying shoelaces. The discomfort and proptosis usually resolve quickly with a head-up posture. Patients often also complain of migraine-like headaches, which can be worse at night. Because the proptosis is intermittent and short-lived, it may take some time for the diagnosis to be made. At rest, with the head up, the eye can in fact look sunken, due to atrophy of the posterior orbital fat caused by the intermittently raised orbital pressure. If the malformation involves the peri-orbital soft tissues or the caruncle, the affected tissues can look purple or engorged (Figure 13.2).

## ARTERIOVENOUS MALFORMATIONS

In the orbit, high-flow lesions can cause venous congestion, raised orbital pressure, and a compartment-type syndrome when the rate of outflow is exceeded by the inflow. Preferential shunting of blood flow through the malformation (arterial steal) can cause ischaemia of the optic nerve, retina, and other orbital tissues. When a high-flow malformation affects the peri-orbital soft tissues, changes such as skin reddening, capillary dilatation, ulceration, and bleeding can occur (Figure 13.3). These can present at any age and are typically progressive, often rapidly so, in and around puberty or pregnancy.

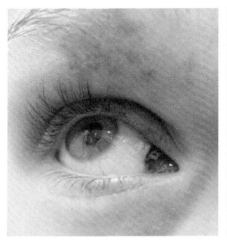
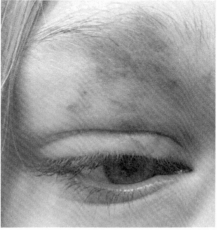

FIGURE 13.2 Child with a venous malformation of the right orbit. The posterior orbital involvement is not clinically apparent at rest, but the malformation is causing purple skin markings of medial upper and lower lid. Note the venous malformation also involves the caruncle and plica.

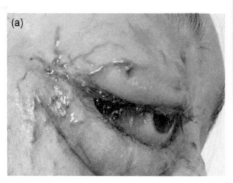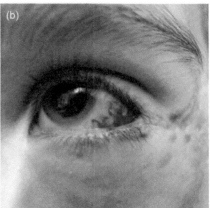

FIGURE 13.3 (a) Right orbital and facial arteriovenous malformation. Note the peri-ocular vascularity, increased bulk of the tissues, chemosis, and injection of the conjunctiva. (b) Left orbital arteriovenous malformation with dilated episcleral and scleral vessels. Note the peri-ocular skin changes.

## Clinical Assessment

The clinical examination should aim to assess the impact of the vascular malformation on:

1) The function of the eye (vision)
2) The structure of the eye, eyelids, and orbit
3) Surrounding tissues, e.g., brain/sinuses

Both the history and examination are essential in forming a differential diagnosis and a management plan; however, these can take place in a more 'free-flowing', less rigid structure compared to that of the adult orbital assessment. Although the technique of paediatric orbital examination is not comprehensively outlined in this chapter, clinical tips are given throughout.

# HISTORY

The presentation can vary greatly with vascular malformations. It is important to establish whether the patient is presenting with an acute event of a known malformation or whether this is the first presentation. These conditions are present since birth, but they can lie 'dormant' within the orbit in the early years, grow with the child, and present later with an acute or acute-on-chronic episode.

All vascular anomalies may have acute events due to thrombosis; pain and inflammation appear to be the most common presenting factors with these events (Figure 13.4).

*Tip*: Ask to see old photographs to illustrate presentation and progression of the clinical picture.

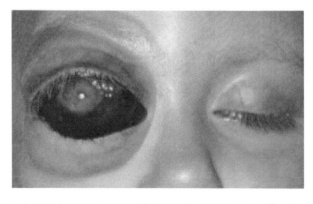

FIGURE 13.4 Acute onset of orbital haemorrhage and inflammation in a patient with right orbital lymphatic malformation. The patient presented with gross proptosis, peri-ocular and subconjunctival haemorrhage, and lagophthalmos. She had optic nerve dysfunction and quickly developed exposure keratitis.

---

### BOX 13.1: POINTS FOR HISTORY TAKING

What are the symptoms and signs? And when did they start? How did they progress? Do they fluctuate?

1) Reduced vision/pain/double vision/change in visual behaviour?
2) Abnormal position of the eye in the orbit? Proptosis or a vertical/horizontal displacement?
3) Swelling/discolouration/bleeding of the eyelid and/or conjunctiva?

Any triggers? Any pre-existing or associated conditions, e.g., viral upper respiratory tract infection? Vaccines? Any pre-existing peri-ocular asymmetry or ocular conditions?

*Tip:* Ask about glasses, patching, and squint.

Any previous changes in eyelid or eye appearance? Any changes with crying/on strenuous activity?

---

# EXAMINATION

This may have to be performed concurrently with the history, depending on the age and mood of the child. The examination parameters are the same for an adult examination but may be more dependent on observation and examination of photographs. In paediatric orbital conditions, there are few hard signs that can definitively differentiate one condition from another, particularly in an acute presentation. However, there may be subtle clues in the examination which lead the diagnosis toward a vascular malformation.

*Tip:* Clinical assessment must be comprehensive, looking at ocular, orbital, and facial signs and symptoms to form a differential diagnosis and guide management decision-making. It is always important to examine the pupils and fundus for optic nerve compromise, even if the lesion is thought to be predominantly only involving the eyelids.

*Tip:* Acute events secondary to thrombosis may cause florid inflammatory signs and symptoms, including pain, and may mimic more common paediatric orbital conditions such as orbital cellulitis.

## ARTERIOVENOUS MALFORMATIONS – CLINICAL CLUES

- Engorged episcleral and scleral vessels, inflammation of the orbital tissues: chemosis and injection of eyelids and conjunctiva (Figure 13.3)
- Raised intra-ocular pressure
- Engorged retinal vessels, disc swelling +/– atrophy (Figure 13.5)

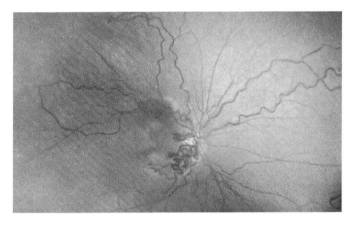

FIGURE 13.5 Photo of posterior pole of the right eye in a child with an arteriovenous malformation of the orbit. Note optic disc atrophy, abnormal vasculature, and retinal pallor.

## VENOUS MALFORMATIONS – CLINICAL CLUES

- Increased vasculature of the peri-ocular tissue. Look in different lighting conditions for increased vasculature around the eyes, forehead, and cheek (Figure 13.2).
- Patients may have subtle enophthalmos due to the orbital fat atrophy. A deep superior sulcus may highlight the presence of enophthalmos.
- Valsalva manoeuvre may make abnormal vasculature, peri-ocular swelling, or eye displacement more obvious.

## LYMPHATIC MALFORMATIONS – CLINICAL CLUES

- There may be no signs other than subtle peri-ocular asymmetry until an acute event occurs.
- Acute events may vary from 'quiet' proptosis (Figure 13.6) to dramatic inflammatory episodes (Figure 13.4). These may involve acute proptosis or bulging of cysts in the peri-ocular tissues.
- Clues in the non-acute phase: proptosis and globe displacement, eyelid swelling with discolouration but not increased vasculature, yellow/pale pink lesions in any of the fornices, and medial canthi, blood-filled cysts (Figure 13.7).
- *Tip:* Even if the LM is confined to the forehead or eyelids, it is still important to examine the orbit and eye and look for occult orbital disease.

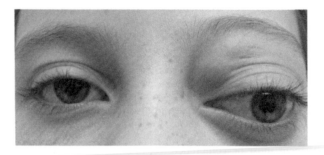

FIGURE 13.6 Previously undiagnosed left orbital lymphatic malformation in a 12-year-old female which presented with acute left proptosis and eyelid swelling. Note the blue tinge overlying the blood-filled cysts in the medial upper lid.

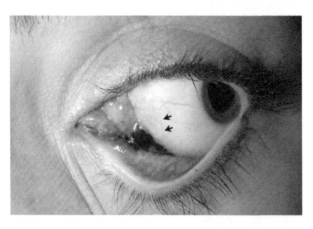

FIGURE 13.7 Black arrows point to small yellow lesions in the episclera. There is old blood within the conjunctiva of the caruncle and inferior fornix (chocolate cysts).

---

### BOX 13.1: SUMMARY OF EXAMINATION

Photographs from different angles may provide valuable insight into the presence of globe displacement. A worm's eye view (from below) is particularly useful for proptosis.

*Tip:* Examining the patient in different lighting conditions may allow features such as vascularity, subtle prominences, and colouring to be observed, e.g., in natural daylight and artificial room light.

---

- Look for 'chocolate cysts' – caused by bleeding into the conjunctiva (Figure 13.7).
- Try to differentiate between bruising versus swelling/infiltration of the lids.
- Are there yellow lesions/cysts involving the medial/lateral canthus?
- It is possible for the disease to mainly involve the 'pre-septal' eyelid tissues and not involve the eye or orbital structures.
- Is the eye pushed forward and/or displaced in other directions, e.g., hypoglobus/ hyperglobus, medial/lateral displacement?

*Tip:* Look for inferior scleral show, i.e., the sclera which is normally hidden behind the lower lid (Figure 13.4).

- Is there limitation of eye movement due to the orbital mass effect?
- Is there yellow discolouration of the medial bulbar conjunctiva (around the plica and semilunaris)? See Figure 13.7.
- Are there conjunctival bleeds (old = brown or fresh = red)?
- Does the lesion become more prominent/more engorged or induce/exacerbate proptosis when the patient performs a Valsalva manoeuvre?

## Eye Exam: Summary

- Does the child object to the other eye being covered?
- Visual acuity reduction (compare to the other eye or baseline).
- Is there an RAPD?
- Colour vision – in an older child.
- Raised intra-ocular pressure with acute event of thrombosis or chronically in congested orbits?
- Optic disc appearance: swollen/not swollen/atrophied?

## ASSESSING RISK OF AMBLYOPIA/VISUAL LOSS

The following are risks to developing amblyopia and must be assessed by an ophthalmologist:

- Ptosis covering the pupil (Figure 13.8). Note that the ptosis not covering the pupil may cause refractive error, so a specialist ophthalmic assessment is still needed.
- Displacement of the globe, in any plane (Figure 13.6).
- Refractive error.
- Squint (secondary to any of the above).
- Raised intra-ocular pressure.
- Exposure keratopathy due to proptosis and/or abnormal corneal wetting.
- Direct or indirect compression of the optic nerve (intra-conal or apical mass, orbital congestion).
- Ischaemia of the ocular structures secondary to shunting of blood.

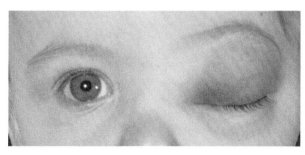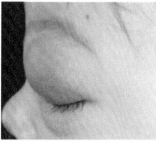

FIGURE 13.8 Left peri-ocular lymphatic malformation, present at birth, with both orbital and eyelid involvement. The lesion was initially diagnosed as a haemangioma, but imaging confirmed a lymphatic malformation. The malformation was predominantly microcystic and treated with serial sclerotherapy procedures.

# IMAGING

Ultrasound (US) of the orbit is quick and relatively straightforward to perform and easy to access for urgent cases. Generally, US and magnetic resonance imaging (MRI) should both be performed at the time of an initial assessment, as they give different, complimentary information. US is well tolerated by most children of any age once you have won their confidence and with the use of distraction techniques. Use a high-resolution small footprint linear probe such as one with a hockey stick configuration and warm the ultrasound jelly. Scanning the brow and then slowly moving onto the upper lid prompts the child to spontaneously close the eye. The globe provides a very useful window into the posterior orbit. Radiologists can relate this approach to the use of a full bladder to scan the pelvis. Scan diagonally through the globe to interrogate the opposite side of the orbit. Transverse views suffice for all areas of the orbit except the roof, where lesions can be missed behind the overhanging superior rim of the orbit. Check the roof of the orbit by scanning in a longitudinal plane while aiming cranially. Alternatively, use a transverse orientation through the lower lid and again tilt the probe cranially. Then change the depth settings to interrogate the medial canthus.

Most MRI departments will have a standard orbital imaging protocol. Fat-saturated T2-weighted sequences are often the most useful, though a range of sequences are required to interrogate suspected thrombus and exclude other pathologies. Diffusion weighted imaging is invaluable if there is any suspicion of a tumour rather than a vascular malformation. Ensure the orbit is imaged in all three planes and that there is at least one whole head sequence in the initial scan to exclude extra-orbital disease or other pathologies. Contrast-enhanced sequences in two planes are essential on initial imaging but may not be required for routine follow-up. MR angiogram (MRA) sequences are only required in cases of suspected high-flow disease.

A computed tomography (CT) angiogram (CTA) is very valuable for high-flow lesions (see below), and CT is useful to look for bone erosion in atypical cases and to provide three-dimensional (3D) reconstruction images in cases that may have caused orbital expansion or remodelling. But otherwise, CT holds limited value other than in an urgent setting when it can be useful to exclude other acute pathologies such as orbital cellulitis until an MRI can be obtained.

## LYMPHATIC MALFORMATIONS: IMAGING FEATURES

Typically, an orbital LM consists of thin-walled macrocysts in the posterior orbit. These can lie intra-conally, extra-conally, or in both spaces and may extend pre-septally. They often contain blood products from new or past intra-lesional bleeds, which manifest as floating debris or fluid-fluid levels (Figure 13.9). A malformation may also include foci of more solid microcystic disease, typically seen in the superficial soft tissues of the medial canthus (Figure 13.10). It is not uncommon for the malformation to be associated with extra-orbital disease in the brow or forehead. As elsewhere, LMs of the orbit demonstrate wall enhancement only on CT and MRI.

In some cases, a posterior orbital malformation is entirely microcystic and presents as a solid mass. These lesions are often a diagnostic dilemma, as they can mimic a solid tumour. Note, too, that sclero-therapy can convert a macrocystic lesion into a more solid microcystic mass, so this appearance can be

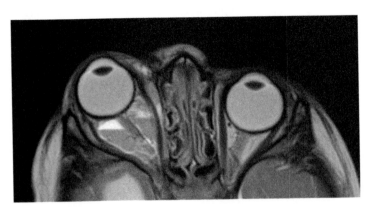

FIGURE 13.9 Axial T2-weighted MRI image showing a fluid-fluid level within several lymphatic cysts in the right retro-orbit. Note the associated severe proptosis. Part of the malformation extends medially into the extra-conal space and into the medial pre-septal tissues.

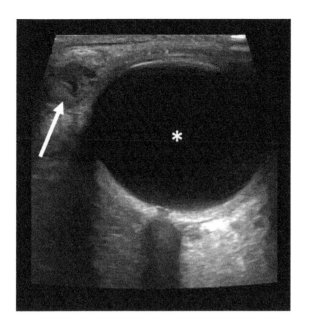

FIGURE 13.10 Axial ultrasound image of the left orbit showing heterogeneity of the soft tissues in the medial canthus (white arrow). The globe is indicated by an asterisk. Note the beautiful detail of the optic disc at the back of the globe and the optic nerve complex extending posteriorly from the disc.

seen after intervention. The stroma of these lesions should enhance to some degree. Organised thrombus in a cyst can be a diagnostic challenge, as it is often difficult to distinguish an organised clot in a lymphatic cyst from a clot in a thrombosed VM. It may be necessary to wait for the lesion to declare itself; as the thrombus resolves, the imaging features and clinical presentation usually become more typical.

# VENOUS MALFORMATIONS: IMAGING FEATURES

VMs of the orbit are easily underestimated with the patient at rest and lying supine. Venous channels often become more obvious with a Valsalva manoeuvre or with the patient sitting up and their head hanging forward. This is an awkward position for ultrasound scanning but can be very helpful diagnostically. For CT or MRI, one should specifically request that part of the scan is done either with an active Valsalva manoeuvre when the child can comply or with the child prone (Figure 13.11). VMs that fluctuate significantly in size with position or effort are more likely to have generous venous outflow from the orbit, and this has significance in terms of treatment planning, so it is worth commenting on in a radiology report. Some VMs are made up of relatively dense, spongiform stroma rather than patulous channels. These can be difficult to differentiate from a microcystic LM or another solid pathology, but they often still change in size to a degree with blood flow and may contain phleboliths. All VMs of the orbit should enhance, but in cases in which inflow is slow, enhancement can be patchy or late and may be seen only on the last sequence of the study.

Subtle associated signs of venous disease in the orbit include a paucity of retroconal fat and involvement of the bone. Look for prominent venous channels along the dura or elsewhere in the adjacent intracranial space.

# ARTERIOVENOUS MALFORMATIONS: IMAGING FEATURES

US demonstrates dilated draining veins which contain arterialised Doppler flow waveforms and hypertrophied feeding arteries. It may be possible to identify nidal architecture at the centre of the lesion. MRI, MRA, and CTA will also show dilated feeding arteries and draining veins with a mesh of nidal vessels. There may be minor changes in vessel calibre or flow with changes in patient position or with a Valsalva manoeuvre.

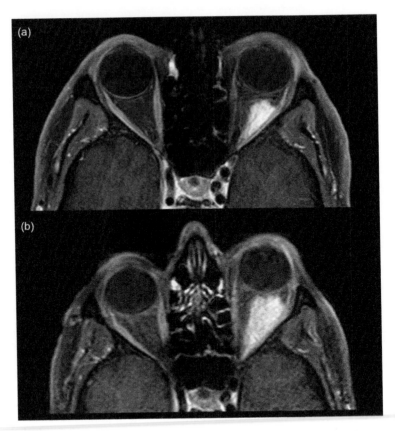

**FIGURE 13.11** Axial T2-weighted MRI images showing a small venous malformation in the lateral aspect of the left intra-conal space. The images were acquired (a) at rest and (b) during a Valsalva manoeuvre. The lesion has increased in size with the resultant increase in venous pressure.

# BIOPSY

Biopsy is very rarely needed but can be considered if the lesion does not fit the expected clinical and/ or radiological profile.

*Clinical suspicions*

- Lesion has an insidious onset of presentation with progressive intra-orbital mass effects, e.g., proptosis, limitations in eye movements, orbital congestion
- Lesion invades surrounding areas over time, e.g., temporalis fossa, intra-nasal cavity, or sinuses
- Lesion is associated with intra-ocular inflammation
- Lesion continues to expand despite sclerotherapy treatment

*Radiological suspicions*

- Destruction of adjacent bone
- Diffusion restriction in MRI sequences
- Homogenous lesions without cysts ('solid' appearance)

## HOW TO BIOPSY

Any open orbital biopsy should be planned carefully to approach the lesion with good visualisation and access. For example:

- Apical and intra-conal lesions may require lateral orbital wall removal and subsequent refixation
- Lateral or orbital-floor based lesions may require a 'swinging-lid' approach (Figure 13.12)
- Anterior superior lesions may be accessed through an upper-lid skin crease approach

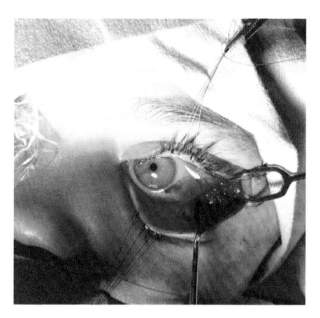

FIGURE 13.12 Biopsy of an inferolateral orbital mass, showing a lower lid, transconjunctival approach with a lateral canthotomy to access the inferior or lateral orbit.

Fine needle aspirate (FNA) and core needle biopsies may be useful in homogenous, superficial orbital lesions; however, the ability to gain haemostasis is limited. Image-guided core needle biopsy of deeper orbital lesions, although less invasive than open biopsy, cannot be considered a 'low risk' procedure due to the risk of orbital bleeding. The risks may be increased with multiple passes required for more heterogenous lesions. Tranexamic acid may be advised for any procedure.

# EMERGENCY MANAGEMENT

All types of vascular malformation may cause acute orbital changes secondary to thrombosis, inflammation, and secondary infection.

The orbit is a closed compartment with a limited capability to accommodate large, sudden changes in mass. Compression near the apex of the orbit can, in turn, cause venous congestion (with further inflammation), compression of the optic nerve, and raised intra-ocular pressure. These patients need to be admitted for an urgent eye examination to assess their optic nerve function.

*Tip:* Globe displacement, eye movement limitation, conjunctival bleeding, chemosis, and signs of optic nerve compromise suggest an intra-orbital event.

Urgent treatment for an orbital vascular malformation would be required for:

1) Ocular surface compromise due to proptosis or chemosis, and/or
2) Optic nerve compromise due to mass effect on the optic nerve

The corneal surface may suffer due to proptosis and exposure or a 'dellen' effect, in which chemosis may cause a localised toxicity and dryness.

## CORNEAL PROTECTION METHODS INCLUDE:

- Topical lubrication and anti-inflammatories
- Lid tarsorrhaphy
- Amniotic membrane graft

## TREATMENT OF OPTIC NERVE COMPROMISE

This usually aims to reduce the mass effect or the sequelae of the mass effect, inflammation, and further bleeding:

1) Lateral canthotomy and cantholysis to reduce the compartment effect (general anaesthetic [GA] recommended)
2) Systemic dexamethasone to reduce inflammation within the orbit
3) Tranexamic acid to reduce the chance of further bleeding
4) Reduce intra-ocular pressure (if elevated) using systemic Diamox™ (acetazolamide)

*Tip:* Open surgical drainage of clots within cysts can cause further bleeding and little real decompression of the orbit. Vascular malformation tissue may also be more prone to infection if a drain is left *in situ*.

The acute events associated with vascular malformations respond to systemic steroids, but most children are usually admitted under the presumptive diagnosis of infective orbital cellulitis, as this is the more common condition, and steroids as a first-line therapy for this diagnosis without initial antibiotics is controversial. If there is a strong suspicion or known diagnosis of an orbital vascular malformation, then it is advisable to start antibiotics, obtain imaging as soon as possible to exclude sinus disease and then commence systemic steroids.

# ORBITAL SCLEROTHERAPY FOR LOW-FLOW MALFORMATIONS

The principles of sclerotherapy are well described in earlier chapters and are the same in the orbit. The significant difference here is that the lesion is in a small, confined space, so every effort must be made to minimise procedure-related swelling. Additionally, the optic nerve lies very close to the site of any posterior orbital intervention. Finally, any venous outflow is to the intracranial vessels, such as the cavernous sinus and dural venous plexuses, and the operator must be very mindful of this when considering where sclerosant drugs may drain. Inadvertent trauma to the ophthalmic artery or its branches could lead to visual loss.

As with malformations in other sites, sclerotherapy is a means of symptom control should not be considered a cure. A significant proportion of patients will require repeat treatments, especially as each intervention in the orbit should be approached with restraint. It is often better to schedule a child for 2–4 cautious procedures than aim to try to get a good result with one aggressive intervention.

The primary aim of orbital sclerotherapy is to shrink the malformation so that it causes less mass effect and is less likely to compromise visual function (3). If visual acuity is affected at presentation, it may improve with a combination of sclerotherapy and active ophthalmological strategies such as patching or refraction, but this is not always the case. Additionally, the soft tissues of the orbit do not always return to their original configuration after an acute event, such as can be seen with a bleed into lymphatic cysts, so cosmetic symmetry is often not entirely regained. It is important to set expectations early with the family in this regard.

After any acute event, sclerotherapy should be delayed, if at all possible, until the orbital inflammation has settled. A quiescent orbit will have a less florid response to sclerotherapy so that the risk of a repeat bleed or significant swelling in the immediate post-operative period is reduced.

Bleomycin is now widely regarded as the sclerosing agent of choice for orbital malformations (4). It tends to cause less swelling and inflammation than other agents, such as sodium tetradecyl sulfate (STS), and reaction to the drug is generally predictable. Importantly, the dose limit in the posterior orbit is 2,000 IU (equivalent to 2 mg or 2 USP units). A small additional dose can be infiltrated pre-septally, with caution, to treat concurrent peri-orbital disease.

---

### BOX 13.3: SCLEROTHERAPY TECHNIQUE

* Perform the procedure in an interventional radiology suite with high quality ultrasound and angiography equipment (ideally biplane).
* General anaesthesia.
* Routine precautions to protect skin and lungs from potential bleomycin effects.

---

- Single dose of dexamethasone on induction.
- Patient positioned supine.
- Preparation of the orbital area with antiseptic povidone-iodine solution, avoiding corneal abrasion.
- US-guided puncture of the largest or most accessible component of the malformation, using a 22G spinal needle or equivalent.
- Puncture through the upper or lower lid, choosing the shortest route and without traversing the path of the optic nerve (Figure 13.13). Make every effort to minimise needle manipulation in the orbit to avoid provocation of a bleed.
- For LMs, aspirate the largest cyst(s) if possible, but do not spend time or effort trying to access every single cyst (see previous point). Send fluid for laboratory analysis if there is any concern regarding the diagnosis or the presence of infection.
- For VMs, an inspiratory breath hold administered by the anaesthetist may briefly increase the size of the malformation and provide a bigger target for puncture.
- Inject a small volume (0.5–1 mL) iodinated contrast medium during biplane digital subtraction angiography to exclude the presence of any vascular connections.
- If there is posterior venous outflow (seen far more commonly with a VM than an LM), occlusion of the outflow could be considered prior to injection of the sclerosant (Figure 13.14). Alternatively, re-position the needle tip and repeat the previous step to try to access a portion of the malformation without venous outflow.
- Inject up to 2,000 IU bleomycin. This can usually be performed under US guidance only to minimise radiation dose to the orbit and allow real-time visualisation of the malformation filling with sclerosant.
- Remove the needle.
- Treat any peri-orbital disease with a small additional dose of bleomycin, under US guidance, using a 23-25G needle.
- Check pupillary reactions for mydriasis (pupillary dilatation) on the treated side.
- Leave eye uncovered to allow regular post-operative assessment for complications.
- Overnight inpatient stay is highly recommended to monitor for complications and administer additional analgesia if required.
- Ensure ward staff perform regular (2–4 hourly) clinical reviews and understand the clinical importance of sudden painful proptosis in the immediate post-operative period, as this may require emergency canthotomy (see below).

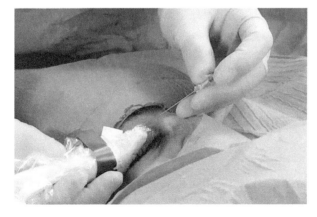

FIGURE 13.13 Photograph of an ultrasound-guided approach to a medial upper-lid puncture using a hockey stick configuration probe and a 22G needle.

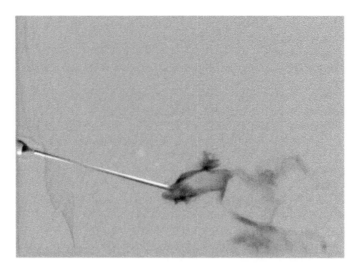

FIGURE 13.14 Lateral digital subtraction angiography image acquired during injection of contrast medium into a posterior orbital malformation. There is flow of contrast posteriorly through both the superior and inferior orbital fissures into the cavernous sinus and pterygoid plexus, respectively.

Intracranial venous outflow from a malformation should be taken seriously. It may reasonably be decided that this precludes percutaneous treatment of the malformation. Alternatively, cautious injection of bleomycin may be justified after re-siting of the needle into a new position which does not lead to any contrast outflow. In experienced hands, embolisation of the venous outflow can be considered (5). In this case, consultation with an interventional neuroradiologist is strongly recommended.

## COMPLICATIONS

Complications of orbital sclerotherapy include visual loss, temporary mydriasis, and swelling or bleeding causing proptosis. Acute proptosis may compromise the optic nerve and is an ophthalmological emergency (see 'Emergency Management' section). After discharge, caregivers must be well informed about the risk of sudden post-operative proptosis and know which team to contact or where to present in an emergency. Peri-orbital swelling and bruising is common and can look concerning – cautious reassurance is key here. Minor subconjunctival haemorrhage or chemosis can occur. Regular analgesia may be required for 24–48 hours. The swelling tends to subside after 1–2 weeks, though any improvement in the size of the malformation may take several more weeks.

## FOLLOW-UP

Repeat sclerotherapy, if required, can usually be scheduled after a 6–8-week interval; repeated imaging between procedures is rarely required. Once a course of sclerotherapy is complete, clinical follow-up is recommended at a minimum of 3 and 12 months. The assessment should include orbital US, which is often sufficient to negate the need for MRI, especially in small children for whom a repeat MRI means a repeat general anaesthetic. Further ophthalmological follow-up is often required beyond that period to monitor or treat associated issues such as amblyopia.

## OUTCOMES

The end point of treatment can be difficult to agree upon and should be discussed with the patient and family or caregivers in advance. There is likely to be a small residual component of the malformation in the posterior orbit, but after a series of sclerotherapy procedures, this is highly likely to represent scar tissue rather than active disease (Figure 13.15) (6). Data are scarce regarding recurrence rates, but in

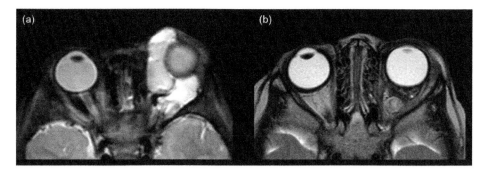

FIGURE 13.15 Axial T2-weighted MRI images before and after serial sclerotherapy. After four procedures: (a) The large macrocystic lymphatic malformation in the left orbit has reduced significantly in size; (b) now, just a small, rounded residual lesion remains at the left orbital apex. Note the improvement in the degree of proptosis.

the authors' experience, symptoms requiring repeat intervention, after the initial series of procedures, occur in 5%–10% of patients.

# EMBOLISATION FOR ARTERIOVENOUS MALFORMATIONS

Choosing a successful and safe treatment strategy for orbital arteriovenous malformations (AVMs) is critically dependent on a clear understanding of the lesion's angio-architecture and its relation to critical structures in the orbit and neighbouring cranial spaces. Generally, the treatment goal should be complete and permanent obliteration of the lesion, and this is usually only achieved through a combination of embolisation followed by surgery (7). A multidisciplinary approach with expert neuroradiology input is vital to avoid diagnostic and management pitfalls.

In cases in which critical structures are intimately involved or there is extra-orbital extension of the AVM niduses into adjacent structures, there may be a role for partial embolisation. Partial targeted embolisation may also be indicated to control acute symptoms such as ulceration, haemorrhage, or raised venous pressure as part of a staged treatment approach.

In addition to non-invasive imaging, transarterial catheter angiogram is essential to confirm the diagnosis and fully understand the angio-architecture before a treatment plan can be formulated. As a minimum, five vessels should be selectively injected (bilateral internal carotid artery [ICA]/external carotid artery [ECA], one vertebral artery) and interpreted by an experienced neuroangiographer.

---

**KEY QUESTIONS**

1. Is there an extra-orbital cause of venous congestion, e.g., carotico-cavernous fistula, cerebral or facial AVM with orbital venous drainage, or anomalous cerebral venous drainage? Unwitting embolisation of orbital vessels can have catastrophic consequences in these conditions (Figure 13.16).
2. What is the arterial supply – ECA vs ICA (ophthalmic), critical arterial boundaries, ECA-ICA anastomoses?
3. What is the AV connection – single-point fistula vs multi-point fistula vs diffuse nidus?
4. What is the venous drainage?

---

Correct assessment will allow an appropriate strategy to be selected (Figure 13.17). Treatment risks will be mitigated by involving an experienced interventional neuroradiologist.

A clear plan of treatment, including realistic assessment of the probability of success, need for staged treatment, and complication risks, should be set out with the patient and caregivers to manage expectations before embarking on any intervention.

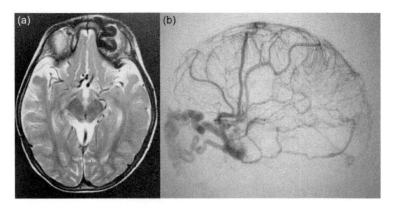

FIGURE 13.16 Pitfall: 10-year-old boy with pulsatile proptosis left eye and (a) dilated vessels on axial T2-weighted MRI sequences, referred as an orbital arteriovenous malformation. Subsequent cerebral catheter angiogram: (b) lateral view of venous phase of selective left internal carotid artery injection demonstrates aplastic transverse sigmoid sinuses with anomalous venous drainage of the entire left hemisphere through dilated left ophthalmic veins. Any disruption to this outflow carries a high risk of subsequent venous infarction in the left cerebral hemisphere.

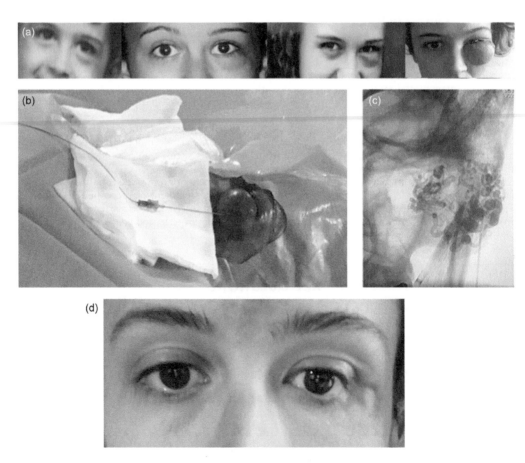

FIGURE 13.17 Left lower lid arteriovenous malformation in a young adult female, showing (a) clinical progression from childhood to young adulthood with rapid enlargement during pregnancy; (b) percutaneous embolisation procedure – the microcatheter is fixed within the 19G needle with a drop of N-butyl cyanoacrylate (NBCA) glue; (c) PHIL™ copolymer embolisation cast visible on an AP unsubtracted fluoroscopic image; (d) the arteriovenous malformation was subsequently completely resected.

**BOX 13.4: TRANSARTERIAL/TRANSVENOUS EMBOLISATION**

Generally transarterial treatments are favoured in the initial stages of treatment with transvenous approaches reserved for later stages.

* General anaesthesia
  * 4 or 5 Fr low-profile femoral arterial or venous sheath
  * 4 or 5 Fr guide catheter advanced to supplying carotid artery/facial vein
  * Systemic heparinisation
* If the transarterial route is chosen
  * Transarterial microcatheter to arteriovenous junction
  * Injection of liquid embolic (e.g., Onyx™, PHIL™) under careful biplane fluoroscopic monitoring
  * Detachable platinum coils or dual lumen neurointerventional micro-balloons (e.g., Scepter™) can be deployed to control flow during the embolic injection
* If the percutaneous route is chosen:
  * Direct puncture of superficial nidal or peri-nidal vessels
  * Controlled injection of liquid embolic agent as above
  * Ensure that the percutaneous needle and any connecting tubing are dimethyl sulphoxide (DMSO)-compatible or they will rapidly degrade and leak during injection

# CHOICE OF EMBOLIC AGENTS

*Traditional liquid sclerosants*
* Ethanol/STS should be generally avoided in orbital high-flow lesions for two reasons – local inflammatory reactions can lead to orbital 'compartment syndrome' and control of venous escape of sclerosant into cerebral or pulmonary vessels can be impossible.

*Copolymers*
* These include non-adhesive liquid embolic agents composed of a biocompatible polymer dissolved in DMSO with a radio-opacifant delivered through a microcatheter under fluoroscopic control. They precipitate on contact with aqueous solution (e.g., blood, water, contrast), flow like lava, and solidify from the outside in as the solvent diffuses away. They deliver in a cohesive manner, forming a spongy, coherent embolus.
* Onyx™/Squid™ are radio-opacified with jet black tantalum powder and can cause permanent skin discolouration in superficial vessels. They can cause sparking with monopolar diathermy during surgery, so surgeons involved in subsequent debulking must be informed.
* PHIL™ is a radio-opacificied agent with faint yellow iodine resulting in no skin discolouration and no risk of diathermy sparking.

# COMPLICATIONS

These include non-target embolisation causing visual loss, stroke, other cranial nerve injury, and skin necrosis.

# FOLLOW-UP

Repeating MRI/MRA imaging of the orbits with the same protocols as the initial study is helpful in staging a response. Repeat catheter angiography may be appropriate to evaluate obliteration of the lesion.

# OUTCOMES

Treatment strategies and, therefore, outcomes are individualised. The most important determinants of 'success' are the extent, location, and angio-architecture of the lesion at outset. Successful obliteration of the shunt(s) is often possible in pre-septal or extra-conal lesions by a carefully planned combined

Outcomes

approach, whereas symptom control is often the realistic goal of more extensive lesions with intra-conal or extra-orbital components.

## SURGERY

Surgical intervention for vascular malformations has become secondary to minimally invasive treatments such as embolisation and sclerotherapy. However, it still has a role.

1) Obtaining biopsies when fine needle aspiration (FNA) or core needle biopsies are not safe or appropriate.
2) Debulking of an AVM post-embolisation.
3) Debulking of a low-flow lesion post-sclerotherapy.
4) Lid repositioning and reconstruction following percutaneous intervention.

Primary surgical excision of active malformations has a higher risk of bleeding both pre- and post-operatively compared to minimally invasive approaches and may also only tackle part of the lesion. LMs can be difficult to excise due to their cystic composition, and residual disease can cause post-operative complications such as infection, lymphatic leaks, and bleeding. Iatrogenic damage to the orbital

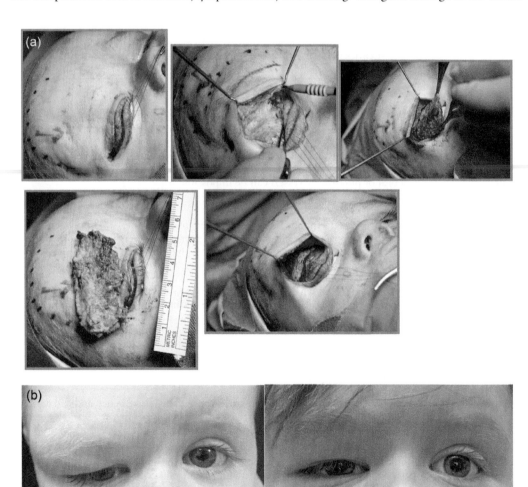

FIGURE 13.18 Excision of right upper-lid lymphatic malformation post-sclerotherapy. (a) The approach was through a skin crease incision. A pre-septal plane was dissected to preserve any functioning levator muscle. A fibrotic sheet of lymphatic malformation was excised down to the superior orbital rim leaving periosteum intact. (b) Pre- and post-surgery photographs. The second photograph was taken prior to subsequent ptosis surgery, which was delayed, as this patient's dormant intra-orbital lymphatic malformation became temporarily symptomatic following an upper respiratory tract infection.

structures during surgery, coupled with residual disease, may cause longer term complications such as intractable pain, diplopia, and disfigurement. However, *after* sclerotherapy or embolisation, vascular malformations may be more amenable to debulking (Figure 13.18).

Aesthetic rehabilitation following minimally invasive treatment methods can be considered on an individual basis. This is dependent on the type of disruption to peri-ocular growth and development, the age of the patient, and the motivation of the patient and the family or caregivers.

# REFERENCES

1. Rootman J, Heran MK, Graeb DA. Vascular malformations of the orbit: Classification and the role of imaging in diagnosis and treatment strategies. *Ophthalmic Plast Reconstr Surg* 2014 Mar–Apr;30(2):91–104.
2. Colletti G, Biglioli F, Poli T, Dessy M, Cucurullo M, et al. Vascular malformations of the orbit (lymphatic, venous, arteriovenous): Diagnosis, management and results. *J Craniomaxillofac Surg* 2019 May;47(5):726–740.
3. De Maria L, De Sanctis P, Tollefson M, Mardini S, Garrity JA, et al. Sclerotherapy for low-flow vascular malformations of the orbital and periocular regions: Systematic review and meta-analysis. *Surv Ophthalmol* 2020 Jan–Feb;65(1):41–47.
4. JA, Hawkins CM, Wojno TH, Jon Kim H. Use of percutaneous bleomycin sclerotherapy for orbital lymphatic malformations. *Hanif AM< Saunders Orbit* 2019 Feb;38(1):30–36.
5. Jin Y, Lin X, Li W, Hu X, Ma G, Wang W. Sclerotherapy after embolization of draining vein: A safe treatment method for venous malformations. *J Vasc Surg* 2008 Jun;47(6):1292–1299.
6. Barnacle AM, Theodorou M, Maling SJ, Abou-Rayyah Y. Sclerotherapy treatment of orbital lymphatic malformations: A large single-centre experience. *Br J Ophthalmol* 2016 Feb;100(2):204–8.
7. Wu CY, Kahana A Immediate reconstruction after combined embolization and resection of orbital arteriovenous malformation. *Ophthalmic Plast ReconstrSurg* 2017 May/Jun;33(3S Suppl 1):S140–S143.

# Intracranial Vascular Malformations

**14**

## Sanjay Bhate, Adam Rennie, and Greg James

## INTRODUCTION AND CLASSIFICATION

Intracranial vascular malformations can be classified depending on the presence or absence of arteriovenous shunting, the vessel type involved, and the location of the lesion. Tumours primarily affecting the vascular tree are rare in children; however, rapidly growing tumours may present with haemorrhage and may mimic ruptured arteriovenous malformations (AVMs).

Most intracranial abnormalities with arteriovenous shunting in the paediatric population are high-flow abnormalities. These can be further classified depending on their angioarchitecture into AVMs and arteriovenous fistulae (AVFs). In the context of an intracranial vascular malformation, an AVF comprises a small number of feeding arteries connected directly to a dilated venous pouch (Figure 14.1), whereas in an AVM, the feeding arteries are connected to the vein via a collection of abnormal nidal vessels without an intervening capillary bed (Figure 14.2). Based on the type of feeding cerebral arteries, intracranial AVMs and AVFs can be categorised as pial or dural.

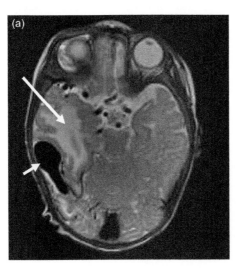
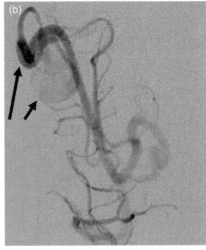

FIGURE 14.1 (a) Axial T2-weighted MRI image showing the large venous sac (short arrow) of an arteriovenous fistula (AVF) with surrounding oedema (long arrow) due to venous hypertension; (b) image from a subsequent catheter angiogram in the same patient showing a large feeding vessel (long arrow) supplying the venous pouch (short arrow). Note this is an early arterial image and the venous pouch has only just started to fill at this stage, so it is only just visible.

DOI: 10.1201/9781003257417-14

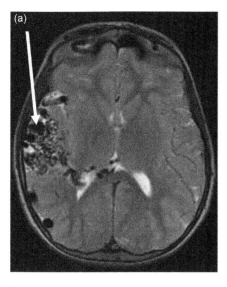

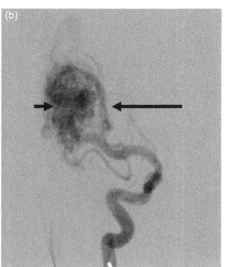

FIGURE 14.2 (a) Axial T2-weighted MRI image of a large arteriovenous malformation (AVM) in the right temporo-parietal region (long arrow); (b) image from a subsequent catheter angiogram in the same patient showing filling of the nidus of the AVM (short arrow) by numerous middle cerebral arterial feeders (long arrow).

Autosomal dominant genetic disorders hereditary haemorrhagic telangiectasia (HHT) and capillary malformation AVM syndrome (CM-AVM) are important genetic causes for extra- and intracranial AVMs (1). Mutations in *ACVRL1* that encodes bone morphogenic protein receptor *ALK1*, and *ENG* that encodes BMP coreceptor endoglin, account for 90% of HHT cases and mutations in *SMAD4* and *GDF2* in the rest. Brain AVMs are found in 10%–30% of HHT patients. Mutations in genes involved in the ephrin pathway, *RASA1* and *EPHB4*, are found in about 30% patients with vein of Galen aneurysmal malformation (VGAM), and *RASA1* and *EPHB4* mutations are found in CM-AVM syndrome. The phenotype in these conditions varies considerably across generations in the same family.

VGAMs and dural sinus malformations (DSMs) are specific types of high-flow arteriovenous shunts that present in the perinatal period (Figures 14.3 and 14.4). VGAM is, in fact, a misnomer, as the malformation is a remnant of the fetal median prosencephalic vein, rather than being the adult great cerebral vein of Galen. Depending on the angioarchitecture of the VGAM, it can be categorised as a mural type in which a small number of feeding arteries connect directly to the venous sac or a choroidal type in which many, usually choroidal, feeding arteries then drain into the venous sac. VGAM should be distinguished from the similarly appearing Vein of Galen aneurysmal dilatation (VGAD), which simply comprises a secondarily dilated vein of Galen due to increased venous outflow from an upstream AVM or AVF.

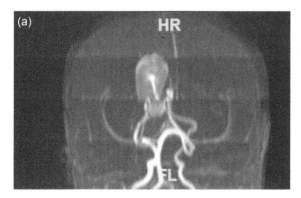

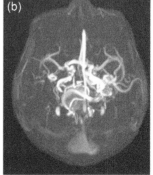

FIGURE 14.3 (a) A time-of-flight (TOF) MRA image showing a vein of Galen malformation (VGAM) of mural type. Note the simple nature of the malformation, with only a few arterial feeders. (b) A TOF MRA image showing a VGAM of choroidal type. In contrast, this type has multiple tortuous arterial feeders.

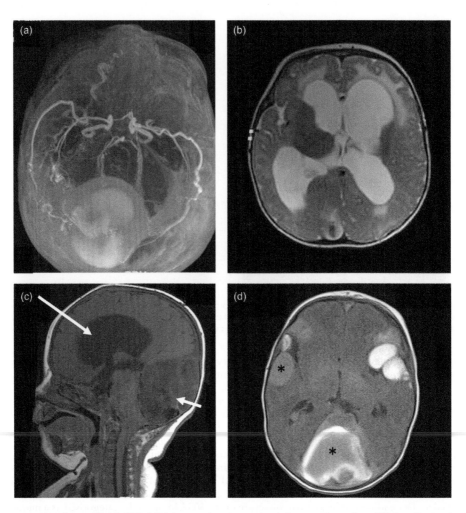

FIGURE 14.4 (a) A time-of-flight (TOF) MRA image showing a dural sinus malformation (DSM), with dural arteries (middle meningeal arteries, predominantly) feeding the malformation; (b) axial T2-weighted MRI image showing acute hydrocephalus secondary to the DSM; (c) sagittal T1-weighted MRI image in the same patient, showing the enormous DSM (short arrow) and dilated ventricles (long arrow); (d) axial T1-weighted MRI image in a different patient showing multiple DSMs with spontaneous thrombosis (asterisk).

Intracranial vascular anomalies with low-flow shunts are rare. Cerebral proliferative angiopathy (CPA) is a poorly understood condition, in which there are nidal vessels, but in comparison with AVMs, they are generally more diffuse and interspersed with normal brain tissue (Figure 14.5). The rate of arteriovenous shunting is slower than in conventional AVMs. Other features of CPA include gliosis within the brain around the malformation, proximal arterial stenosis, and more frequent presentation with seizures rather than haemorrhage.

Intracranial vascular abnormalities without arteriovenous shunting include developmental venous anomalies (DVAs). DVAs are the most common intracranial vascular anomalies, estimated to occur in 3% of the general population. DVAs are abnormal dilated venous structures, often reflecting abnormal venous development in fetal life, but they provide venous drainage to normal brain tissue (Figure 14.6). The imaging appearances are characteristic and often described as *caput medusa*, which comprises radially oriented veins draining into a dilated central venous structure. DVAs are sometimes seen in association with cavernomas and other developmental anomalies of the venous system such as Sturge–Weber syndrome and blue rubber bleb syndrome. DVAs may be found in association with sinus pericranii, which are prominent trans-osseous connections between the intracranial veins and the veins of the scalp or face (Figure 14.7). DVAs are most often detected incidentally on neuroimaging, and although there are case reports and small series describing bleeding, their true incidence is unknown.

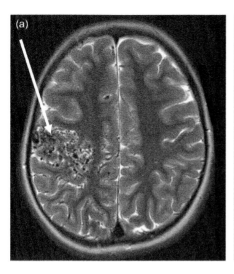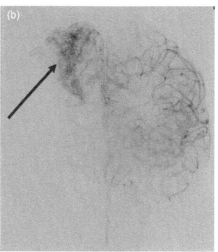

FIGURE 14.5 (a) Axial T2-weighted MRI image and (b) AP digital subtracted angiogram (DSA) image of a patient with proliferative angiopathy (CPA), showing diffuse areas of slow shunting (arrow). There is no true nidus.

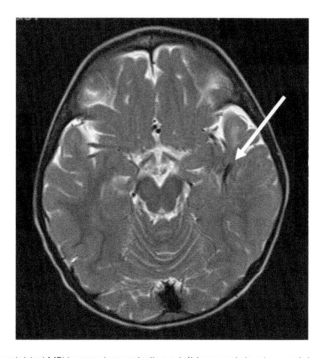

FIGURE 14.6 Axial T2-weighted MRI image demonstrating a left temporal developmental venous anomaly (DVA) (arrow).

In Sturge–Weber syndrome, there is abnormal venous architecture affecting the ipsilateral cerebral hemisphere in association with a capillary malformation (specifically a port-wine stain) of the face (see Chapter 7) (Figures 14.8 and 14.9).

The International Society for the Study of Vascular Anomalies (ISSVA) histological classification is valid for all body sites, including the intracranial lesions; however, historic terminology is often used. For example, cavernomas or cavernous angiomas are also known as cavernous capillary malformations (CCM) and are the second most common of the intracranial vascular anomalies. These are collections

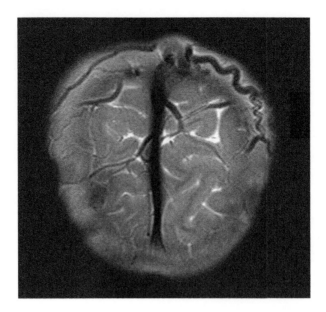

FIGURE 14.7 Axial T2-weighted MRI image at the vertex of a child's head, demonstrating sinus pericranii and multiple venous channels over the scalp.

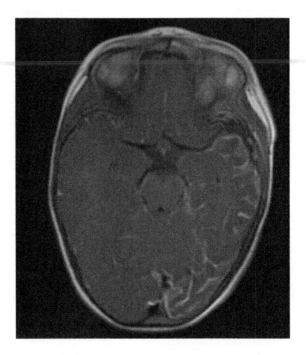

FIGURE 14.8 Contrast-enhanced axial T1-weighted MRI image in a child with Sturge–Weber syndrome. There is widespread enhancement of the pial membrane on the left side of the brain, in keeping with a pial angioma. Note there is also associated parenchymal atrophy on that side.

of thin-walled abnormal capillaries without intervening brain tissue. They are often surrounded by a ring of hemosiderin reflecting microhaemorrhages from the leaky capillaries. These can be single or multiple. Multiple cavernomas are seen in sssfamilial cases. The familial cases show mutations in one of three genes: *KRIT1, CCM2, or PDCD10.* The protein products form a heterodimeric complex that dampens down the activity of kinase MEKK3 that stimulates vessel growth.

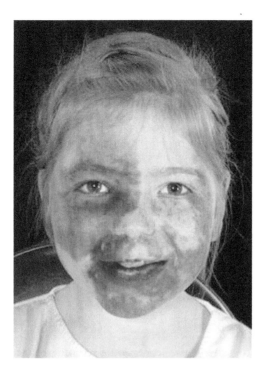

FIGURE 14.9 A child with the characteristic capillary malformation associated with Sturge–Weber syndrome.

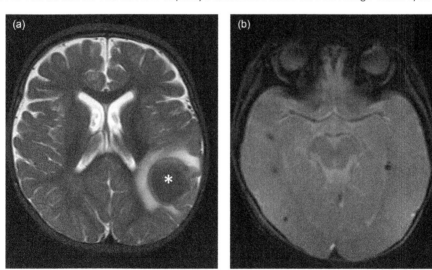

FIGURE 14.10 (a) Axial T2-weighted MRI image of a giant single cavernoma (asterisk) in an infant with surrounding oedema following a significant, recent bleed; (b) an axial gradient echo (GE) sequence MRI image of a different patient demonstrating multiple cavernomas in a familial case. On this sequence, the cavernomas show up as small dark lesions within the pale grey parenchyma.

## CLINICAL PRESENTATION

VGAMs and DSMs can be detected in late pregnancy ultrasound scans but are often undiagnosed at birth. Neonates with torrential arteriovenous shunts may appear normal at birth but then present at 48–72 hours with severe high-output cardiac failure. It is important to consider the diagnosis of VGAM in neonates presenting with unexplained heart failure and pulmonary hypertension. A bruit can often be heard over the cranium, and a simple cranial ultrasound scan is almost always diagnostic.

Children with less severe shunts develop venous hypertension over time and can present in infancy or early childhood with macrocephaly, motor delay, papilloedema, hydrocephalus, and prominent facial veins. Some patients may only have macrocephaly and prominent facial veins, and the diagnosis is established incidentally after neuroimaging is carried out for some other purpose, e.g., after a head injury. Exceptionally, patients may present in adult life with an intracranial haemorrhage. Although a rare cause, it is important to consider VGAM in the differential diagnosis in young children with large heads and carry out appropriate neuroimaging.

The most common reason for an intracranial vascular malformation of any type to be diagnosed in childhood is when one is detected after a haemorrhagic stroke. A study from our institution reviewing 93 consecutive cases of paediatric haemorrhagic stroke found an underlying vascular malformation in the majority (68/93), of which most were brain AVMs (48/68). This is a different situation from that seen in adults, for which the most common cause of spontaneous intracranial haemorrhage is aneurysm rupture. Children with haemorrhagic stroke present with sudden onset of headache, seizures, a reduced level of consciousness, and neurological deficits. These patients require urgent neurosurgical evaluation and appropriate intervention.

Cavernomas can present with intracranial haemorrhage as well, but a massive intracranial haemorrhage due to a cavernoma is rare (Figure 14.10). Other presentations of an intracranial vascular malformation are seizures, steal symptoms due to re-routing of blood from normal tissue (such as headaches or intermittent neurological deficits), or increasingly, incidental findings on neurological imaging performed for unrelated reasons. Of AVMs, 20%–30% are detected incidentally after imaging is done for non-specific symptoms such as headache or following head injury. AVMs and cavernomas can also present with focal seizures without obvious haemorrhage. Refractory focal seizures and progressive hemiplegia are a hallmark of Sturge–Weber syndrome. Patients with CPA almost always present with seizures or a neurological deficit without haemorrhage.

## CLINICAL ASSESSMENT

VGAM and DSM should be considered in babies presenting with unexplained cardiac failure. Intracranial haemorrhage is the cardinal symptom of children with AVMs and cavernomas.

In children who do not present acutely, symptoms and signs may relate to intracranial venous hypertension. The patients may have motor delay, a large head, and/or prominent veins on the face. There may be a history of epistaxis. Patients with AVM and cavernomas may present with seizures. Headache is not a specific symptom but may lead to imaging and detection of asymptomatic lesions. Focal neurological deficits and visual symptoms are rarely reported as presenting features.

A family history of epistaxis and intracranial haemorrhage should be sought, as these may be clues to the underlying genetic cause.

Examination should include measurement of head circumference and tracking of head growth on appropriate centile charts. The child's skin should be examined for the presence of telangiectasia and other vascular marks (Figure 14.11, 14.12). A full neurological examination, including assessment

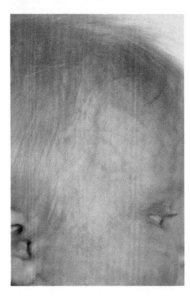

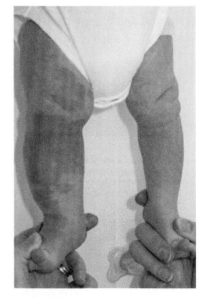

FIGURE 14.11 A young child with an underlying intracranial shunt, demonstrating macrocephaly and enlarged facial veins.

FIGURE 14.12 A child with CM-AVM of the right lower limb.

for acuity papilledema and visual fields, should be carried out to assess the impact of the vascular malformation.

# IMAGING

Cranial ultrasound is very useful to detect vascular malformations in neonates and very young infants when the anterior fontanelle is still open (Figure 14.13). However, to establish a definitive diagnosis, one or multiple modalities of neuroimaging such as computed tomography (CT), CT angiography (CTA), magnetic resonance imaging (MRI), MR angiography (MRA), and catheter angiography is essential.

CT and CTA are very useful in the acute setting when patients present with acute intracranial haemorrhage. It is widely available, quick and accurate, and, therefore, universally used to guide immediate neurosurgical management.

MRI provides definitive information about the brain parenchyma and, when combined with MRA, is often diagnostic. MRI is essential to assess the impact of the vascular malformation as well as plan potential treatments. Cavernomas are seen on MRI as lobulated structures surrounded by a rim of hemosiderin; blood-sensitive sequences, such as gradient echo or susceptibility weighting imaging, are essential to detect tiny multiple cavernomas in familial cases. The main disadvantage of MRI is that it may not be available in an acute setting and requires sedation or general aesthetic to obtain good quality images in young children. It does, however, give vital information about the brain parenchyma, e.g., ischaemia which is important for deciding on optimal management.

Catheter angiography is the gold standard investigation to characterise vascular abnormalities and is the only test that can definitively demonstrate the presence of arteriovenous shunting. Angiography is invasive, requires a general anaesthetic in all children, and should only be carried out by suitably trained interventional neuroradiologists. Procedural complications are rare but include local bruising and hematoma at the site of femoral puncture (5%), stroke due to damage to cerebral arteries (1%), and damage to the femoral artery leading to thrombosis and vascular compromise of the leg (<1%). The dose of contrast medium required may sometimes be a concern, particularly in small children with impaired renal function. In neonates and infants, diagnostic angiography is generally only undertaken as part of definitive endovascular treatment, but in older children, evaluation using angiography is an essential component of the child's diagnostic work-up.

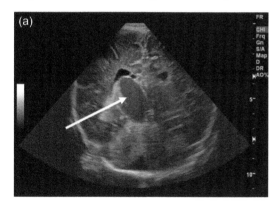 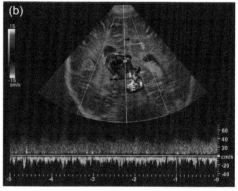

FIGURE 14.13 (a) A coronal cranial ultrasound image in a newborn with cardiac failure, revealing a VGAM which is seen as a large dilated vascular structure near the midline (arrow); (b) a Doppler ultrasound image in the same patient confirming arterialised flow in the VGAM sac.

# EMBOLISATION

Interventional neuroradiologists play a key role in the diagnosis and treatment of vascular malformations in children but should do so within the setting of a wider multidisciplinary team. Ideally, the team comprises neurologists, neurosurgeons, intensivists, anaesthetists, and cardiologists in addition to the neuroradiologist. The team is vital in reaching correct management decisions in this highly complex patient group. In neonates with high-flow shunts, the treatment risks and potential benefits are particularly finely balanced. Furthermore, the development of endovascular techniques has advanced significantly in recent years, as investment in products has led to better endovascular devices and extended what is now possible endovascularly. The endovascular management of three specific conditions is discussed here: namely VGAM, pial AVFs, and DSMs.

## VEIN OF GALEN MALFORMATION

Endovascular treatment is the mainstay of treatment of VGAMs with trans-arterial routes most commonly utilised, although trans-venous or combined approaches have been advocated by some operators. The aim is to occlude the arterial feeders into the venous sac, without impairing arterial blood supply to normal brain or the venous drainage of normal brain/untreated arteriovenous shunt. The presence or absence of normal venous drainage into the sac is difficult to ascertain in the high-flow situation but is a key aspect in determining outcome. Embolisation can be performed with varying concentrations of Histoacryl glue (mixed with Lipiodol [ethiodised oil] and tantalum for increased opacification), coils, and/or copolymer liquid embolics such as Onyx™. Treatment is often staged to allow gradual remodelling of the anatomy.

In a high-output cardiac failure setting, the aim of intervention is to treat the malformation enough to reduce the heart failure and allow the baby to thrive. Should a newborn have heart failure that is either very mild or controlled by oral diuretics, then treatment is delayed, ideally until 3 months of age. Once embolisation treatments are commenced, the timing of the following treatment is agreed by team consensus, aiming at around 3-month intervals, but expedited should there be clinical concern such as developing hydrocephalus or failure to thrive. The issue of proliferation of a network of arterial feeders occurs occasionally and may lead to a situation in which the operators are unable to cure the lesion endovascularly without incurring unacceptable risk. Should the child be developing normally, these partially treated malformations are followed closely both clinically and radiologically.

In children who present at an older age with venous hypertension, embolisation remains the mainstay of treatment. The goal is to reduce the degree of arteriovenous shunting and, thereby, reduce the venous pressure of the cerebral veins, stabilising the child's clinical situation. Occasionally, the enlarged VGAM venous sac causes mechanical obstruction by compression of the tectal plate and aqueduct of Sylvius. In such cases, prompt third ventriculostomy may be required after the embolisation. Usually, low molecular weight heparin is required after embolisation in children with venous hypertension, with the aim of controlling thrombosis of the sac and draining venous sinuses and, hence, preserving any venous drainage of the brain and arteriovenous shunt and reducing venous pressure.

## PIAL ARTERIOVENOUS FISTULA

Treatment of pial AVFs is usually acute (as presenting with heart failure or venous hypertension), with similar treatment devices and methodologies to that described for VGAMs. Whilst the arteriovenous junctions should be targeted, occlusion of the venous sac may be required on later treatments, as occasionally further neovascularity develops around the initial embolisation/feeding artery targets. Long-term cross-sectional follow-up is advised.

## DURAL SINUS MALFORMATION

These vascular malformations can be very large, with every potential dural artery supplying the arteriovenous shunt. The mass effect can be considerable, with a large sac causing distortion of the brain as well as venous congestion. There is usually some thrombus already present within larger malformations. The treatment strategy involves progressive embolisation of the arterial feeders, gradually remodelling the sac, which may be required for normal venous drainage of the brain. Once again, a combination of coil and liquid embolic agents are usually required to achieve occlusion. Low molecular weight heparin is usually administered between treatments to control thrombosis and allow preservation of normal brain venous pathways.

# SURGERY

## AVM

In contrast to the clinical scenario in adults, AVM rupture is a prominent cause of haemorrhagic stroke in children. In addition, many unruptured AVMs are detected on imaging for seizures, other neurological symptoms, or completely incidentally. There is consensus amongst neurosurgeons that ruptured brain AVMs should be treated, as the risk of re-bleeding is significant (except for a small number of lesions in exquisitely eloquent locations which may need to be managed conservatively). For unruptured AVMs, the decision-making is more difficult, as all treatments carry a significant risk of complication, which must be balanced against the uncertain natural history. The ARUBA study attempted to answer this question – a randomised, non-blinded trial in which patients (adults and children) with unruptured brain AVMs were assigned to medical (i.e., no surgery, embolisation, or radiosurgery) or interventional arms (2). The trial found that the risk of death or stroke was significantly less in the medical group at

33 months. Many have interpreted this trial as saying that unruptured AVMs should never be treated. However, there are many criticisms of the trial, most importantly that the short follow-up period (33 months) was insufficient, as the aim of treatment is lifelong obliteration of bleeding risk. This is especially important in paediatric practice, as successful cure of a brain AVM in childhood offers lifelong freedom from the risk of haemorrhage. Research from Boston Children's Hospital suggests that children with brain AVMs managed in a high-volume, specialised centre do well with aggressive treatment, even in unruptured cases (3).

Intracranial AVMs are heterogeneous in their location, size, and angioarchitecture. Each lesion must be considered on its individual merits. To aid neurosurgeons in decision-making, several scoring systems have been developed, the most well-known of which is the Spetzler–Martin grade (4). This grade, which is based on the size, site, and venous drainage of an AVM, ranges from 1 to 5 and predicts the risk of post-surgical neurological deficit. Grades 1 and 2 are so-called 'low-grade AVMs' and are deemed suitable for safe microsurgical excision. Grades 4 and 5 (high-grade AVMs) are usually best treated via other interventions (including multimodality treatment). Grade 3 lesions are a difficult group with regard to decision-making and often require considerable analysis and multidisciplinary debate. A further grading system (the Lawton–Young classification [5]) has been developed to aid decision-making for these 'borderline' (and common) lesions; it factors in age, previous bleeding events, and the anatomical configuration of the nidus. Ultimately, decision-making for treatment of brain AVMs in children is best undertaken in a dedicated multidisciplinary meeting, including neurosurgeons, neurologists, neuro-interventional radiologists, and stereotactic radiosurgeons who can assess each case on its individual merits, followed by discussion with the family and child/young person to make a final plan. It is our experience that several meetings are sometimes required before making a definitive treatment decision, especially in unruptured and/or borderline grade cases.

The decision-making process can be broken up into two stages – first, whether to treat the lesion at all (usually a straightforward decision in ruptured AVMs, but more difficult in unruptured cases), followed by a further discussion, if the decision is to treat, regarding which modality (or modalities) are best. The three tools available to the neurovascular multidisciplinary team are microsurgical resection, embolisation, and stereotactic radiosurgery (Figure 14.14).

Microsurgical resection has the attractive advantage of offering an immediate and long-term cure. However, of the three options, it is the most invasive, requiring a craniotomy and dissection of both

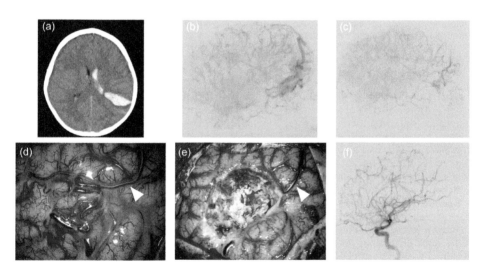

FIGURE 14.14 Case showing multimodality management of a ruptured parietal AVM. A previously well 8-year-old girl presented following a severe sudden onset of headache at school. (a) CT scan showed spontaneous intracerebral and intraventricular haemorrhage on the left. As she remained fully conscious, she was acutely managed non-operatively on the neurosurgical high dependency unit. (b) Catheter angiogram confirmed an underlying AVM. She was referred for stereotactic radiosurgery (SRS). (c) Five years post-SRS, a follow-up angiogram demonstrated significant reduction of the nidus but still some residual arteriovenous shunting. The multidisciplinary team decision was to proceed to craniotomy for microsurgical resection. (d) Intraoperative image demonstrating the AVM nidus on the cortical surface. Note the arterialised vein (arrowhead). (e) Intraoperative image at the end of resection. Note the previously arterialised vein has become a normal dark red colour (arrowhead). (f) Post-operative angiogram confirms successful resection of the nidus. The girl remains well 2 years post-operatively with no new neurological deficits. She has, however, had significant emotional problems relating to her original bleed, requiring psychological support.

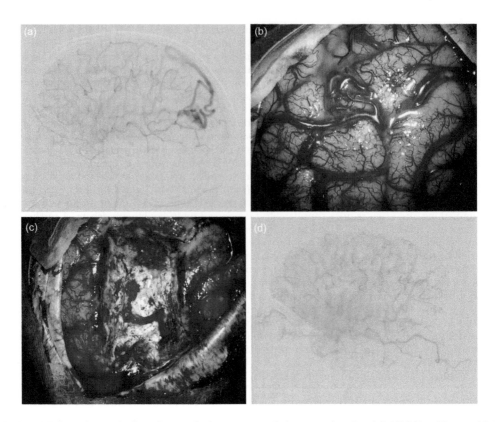

FIGURE 14.15 Case demonstrating microsurgical management of an unruptured parietal AVM in a 15-year-old girl. The patient presented with a history of headache and chronic fatigue syndrome. She underwent an MRI scan, and an unruptured intracranial AVM was discovered. (a) Preoperative angiogram demonstrating a low-grade parietal AVM. Following discussion of the options, including the possibility of conservative management (as this was an unruptured lesion), the young lady opted for surgical treatment (stereotactic radiosurgery was also offered). (b) Intraoperative image demonstrating the AVM nidus on the cortical surface. (c) AVM resection cavity. (d) Post-operative angiogram demonstrating cure. Three years later, she remains well.

the nidus and the associated feeding and draining vessels from the underlying or surrounding brain parenchyma (Figure 14.15). Intracranial AVM surgery is technically challenging, and most units will use adjuncts to improve efficacy and safety, including image-guidance, use of intraoperative fluorescence angiography (with indocyanine green), Doppler ultrasound, and sometimes neurophysiological mapping and intraoperative imaging such as MRI or MRA. Historically, a post-operative angiogram showing no residual arteriovenous shunting was regarded as a permanent cure. However, there is accumulating evidence, especially in children, of late recurrence of 'cured' brain AVMs; follow-up imaging is now recommended (6).

Endovascular embolisation is discussed in the section above. It has two distinct roles in the management of intracranial AVMs. The first is embolisation with curative intent offered as stand-alone treatment; this has the advantage of being less invasive than craniotomy, but evidence exists of higher recurrence rates in the long term (7). The second role is as an adjunct to surgery with preoperative embolisation of feeding arteries. This reduces flow through the nidus of the AVM during surgery, aiming for improved operating conditions and reduced risk to the child. It has the additional advantage of helping with identification of the feeding arteries during the initial dissection, as the embolic material can be visualised with the microscope and ultrasound.

Stereotactic radiosurgery (SRS), such as gamma knife, is an attractive option for many intracranial AVMs. SRS uses collimation (in gamma knife) or a linear accelerator (in other platforms) to deliver high doses of radiation to a lesion with relative sparing of the surrounding brain. In intracranial AVMs, this causes progressive endothelial hyperplasia and gradual 'shrinking' of the nidus, resulting in complete obliteration of the arteriovenous shunt in many cases. The advantage of this technique is its minimally invasive nature; other than the application of a stereotactic frame and the need for repeat diagnostic angiography and an MRI scan on the day of treatment, there are no incisions or cannulation of intracranial vessels. In children, it is our practice to undertake gamma knife SRS under general anaesthesia, although it can be carried out awake (using local anaesthesia for the frame application and angiogram) in older young people and adults. The risk of neurological complications on the day of treatment is negligible (particularly when compared to the substantial risks during microsurgery or embolisation). The disadvantage is that SRS can take up to 5 years to have its effect – during which, the child remains at risk of bleeding and of late side effects such as cerebral oedema or thrombosis. The utility of SRS is limited by lesion size and location; the side effects of radiation are related to both. For large AVMs, staged or multiple treatments are sometimes used (8).

Finally, especially for higher grade lesions, multimodality treatment may be an option. For example, a nidus too large for conventional SRS may be 'pruned' with judicious embolisation to reduce the volume of the lesion to a treatable size. We have used SRS to deal with small post-surgical residual nidus (and vice versa).

## CAVERNOMA

Unlike aneurysms and AVMs, cavernomas are low-flow lesions, and surgical excision is comparatively straightforward, dependent on their location within the brain. In addition, as they are angiographically occult, endovascular treatment is not an option. SRS has been used for cavernoma, but the success of this procedure for these lesions remains controversial.

Despite their attractiveness as surgical targets, the decision on whether to undertake resection of a particular cavernoma can be difficult. Unlike the often-devastating haemorrhagic stroke seen following aneurysm or AVM rupture, cavernoma bleeds are commonly minimally symptomatic, and neurological recovery is usually complete. The natural history is not well understood, and cavernomas may be quiescent for many years after a bleed. Because of this uncertainty, a randomised controlled trial (CARE) is being piloted in the United Kingdom, which is recruiting both adults and children (9). In the absence of Level 1 evidence, currently, most neurosurgeons will consider treatment for surgical accessible lesions which have had at least one clinical bleed, preferring to monitor those patients with asymptomatic or deep cavernomas. In children, many cases will be related to familial multiple cavernomas, a syndrome which is autosomally inherited, so resection of a single lesion is non-curative, in any case, and, therefore, reserved for those that have multiple proven bleeds (10). Finally, some children with cavernomas will develop intractable epilepsy and be managed by an epilepsy multidisciplinary team.

Microsurgical removal of a cavernoma is undertaken via craniotomy (Figure 14.16). Image-guidance and intraoperative ultrasound are often used to aid localisation and to avoid critical structures, sometimes supplemented with neurophysiological mapping. There is often a clear plane of dissection between the lesion and the surrounding brain, often containing old blood products, which can aid the surgeon in achieving complete removal. For those operations undertaken for intractable epilepsy, it is often necessary to resect the so-called 'haemosiderin ring' of chronically injured brain adjacent to the cavernoma itself. Recurrence after complete resection is rare but is seen more often in children with familial multiple cavernoma syndrome. Recurrent lesions can be re-operated or monitored, depending on the clinical scenario.

Brainstem cavernomas require special consideration; there is some evidence that these lesions are particularly symptomatic. Surgical treatment is limited by the exquisite eloquence of the surrounding neural tissue; whilst several 'safe corridors' for surgical access to deep-seated brainstem lesions have

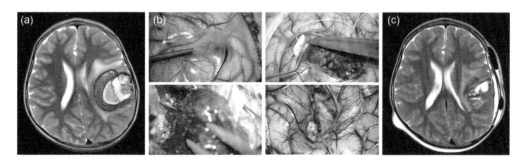

FIGURE 14.16 Case demonstrating surgical management of a left parietal cavernoma. A 3-year-old boy presented with a seizure and new right sided hemiparesis. There was a family history of CCM1 (KRIT1) mutation. (a) MRI demonstrated a large left parietal cavernoma with mass effect. Multiple other small cavernomas were present, consistent with an underlying diagnosis of CCM1. The child was initially managed conservatively but remained symptomatic with evidence of ongoing mass effect and further bleeding on follow-up MRI. Therefore, after multidisciplinary team discussion, the family were offered surgery, which they accepted. (b) Sequential intraoperative images demonstrating the haemosiderin stained cortex and dissection of the cavernoma, with a clear cavity at the end, confirmed on (c) post-operative MRI. The child's neurological deficit resolved. His other lesions were monitored with serial scans, and he was referred to a clinical genetics team for confirmation of an underlying genetic diagnosis.

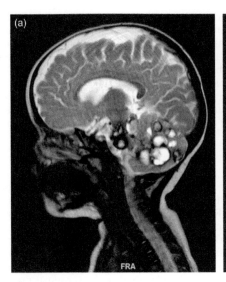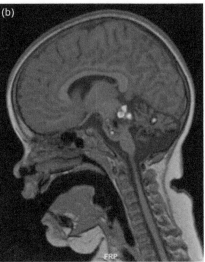

FIGURE 14.17 Case demonstrating non-surgical management of a brainstem cavernoma. A 3-month-old infant presented with bacterial meningitis and underwent neuroimaging prior to lumbar puncture. (a) The sagittal MRI image demonstrates an incidental finding of an extensive posterior fossa cavernoma infiltrating the pons, midbrain, and cerebellum. The lesion's highly eloquent location meant the risks of surgery were extremely high, and the child was managed non-operatively with clinical and radiological surveillance. Genetic analysis confirmed CCM1 (KRIT1 mutation). It became clear over the next 2 years that the child was having multiple symptomatic bleeds. Following discussion with the vascular anomalies multidisciplinary team, she was started on sirolimus. This resulted in a period of clinical and radiological stability which persisted for several years. She is now in mainstream school and thriving at age 8, although she has developed some spastic weakness of the lower extremities. (b) MRI at age 8 demonstrating quiescent cavernomata.

been described, operative morbidity remains considerable even in the most skilled hands. Therefore, consideration is given to non-operative treatment or the use of alternative modalities such as SRS or even chemotherapeutic agents such as sirolimus (Figure 14.17).

## Rationale of Neurosurgical Management

For children presenting with haemorrhagic stroke resulting from bleeding from an intracranial vascular malformation, the acute management strategy is supportive. Many children will have a depressed conscious level and will require intubation for airway protection. Acute imaging in the form of a CT scan is usually performed at presentation due to suspicion of an intracranial bleed. If blood is seen on the scan, we recommend immediate progression to obtaining a CTA, which is a critical investigation to reveal any underlying high-flow lesion, such as an aneurysm or AVM, which will inform immediate neurosurgical management decisions. Such patients should be transferred emergently to a paediatric neurosciences centre and admitted to an intensive care or high dependency bed. Those children with raised intracranial pressure (ICP), i.e., those with a depressed consciousness and/or pupillary dilatation, should be operated on immediately to relieve pressure. Generally, attempting to remove all of the blood clot is not advised, as it can precipitate further bleeding from the underlying lesion, and the cavity left by the resorbed clot can facilitate later microsurgery. An external ventricular drain, decompressive ICP, and, for those children who are predicted to require ongoing ventilation and sedation, an ICP monitor are inserted.

If an AVM is thought to be the cause of the bleed, the risk/balance analysis favours careful evaluation. We usually recommend obtaining a catheter angiogram within the first 48 hours of the bleed to confirm the diagnosis and to assess for so-called 'high-risk features', such as perinidal aneurysms or venous varices. If the latter are detected, and it is thought safe to do so, selective embolisation of these 'weak points' may be undertaken. Curative embolisation is not recommended at this stage, as the risk of complications are high and the early re-bleed risk is low. We then let the child recover and rehabilitate before undertaking a further suite of investigations (repeat CTA, MRI, and catheter angiogram) at 6–8 weeks after the ictus to fully delineate the AVM once the acute clot and swelling have resolved, followed by discussion of the options in a neurovascular multidisciplinary meeting to plan definitive management as discussed in the section above.

Finally, bleeds from cavernomas only rarely present with a child in extremis. More often, the situation is a patient with a headache or having had a single seizure. This allows time to admit the child for detailed neurological assessment, appropriate imaging (MRI), and discussion of management with the family. For those rare bleeds which cause significant ongoing mass effect (such as prolonged headaches or alteration of consciousness level), early surgery (within the first 14 days after ictus) has the advantage that the cavernoma is often surrounded by liquid clot, making dissection straightforward; however, the swollen and friable nature of the brain so soon after the bleed may make identification and resection of the entire cavernoma more difficult, increasing the risk of residual lesion. For this reason, cavernoma surgery is often undertaken on a planned elective basis.

## Complications of Surgical Treatment

Neurovascular surgery is regarded as the most technically challenging and high-risk subspecialty of neurosurgery, and the potential complications are significant. The most critical complications involve injury to blood vessels or brain tissue during surgery, resulting in permanent neurological deficits or even death. As neurovascular malformations are intimately related to normal blood vessels, these risks are often present. Intraoperative rupture of lesions such as AVMs can be very dangerous, as their arterial supply means the entire surgical field will become obscured very quickly, and, particularly in children, hypovolaemia can ensue within seconds. Therefore, a strategy should be decided prior to commencing dissection of the lesion on how to deal with this situation should it arise, including obtaining proximal control and keeping the field clear of blood. The surgeon must remain cool and not reflexively occlude critical blood vessels, resulting in a potentially devastating stroke. Communication and planning with the anaesthetic and nursing teams are critical to optimising brain perfusion during this period. Sometimes strategies such as circulatory arrest with adenosine or suppression of cerebral metabolism with barbiturates are required to permit periods of occlusion or manipulation.

Due to these risks, the consent process for neurovascular surgery must be particularly robust. We advocate clear and consistent communication with families, including frank discussion of the advantages and disadvantages of surgery and explanation of the risks, with reference to local institutional series and statistics. Building trust and understanding with families and children may take multiple consultations and often involve the support of specialist nurses and play therapists.

# OUTCOMES AND FOLLOW-UP

Despite the dramatic possible complications described above, the majority of children with intracranial vascular malformations have a good long-term prognosis. It is important that all children and young people have robust clinical and radiological follow-up planned and arranged and that radiological investigations are reviewed in a neurovascular multidisciplinary context. As well as the clinical follow-up, it is increasingly recognised that children and young people who have suffered haemorrhagic stroke, even without overt neurological deficit, may suffer neuropsychological and emotional adverse effects in the long term. In addition, many will have more specific neurological deficits (such as spasticity) or epilepsy after a bleed. Therefore, the treatment team following the child should include paediatric neurologists, specialist nurses, and neuropsychologists in addition to a neurosurgeon and interventional neuroradiologist.

## KEY MESSAGES

* Intracranial vascular malformations can be subdivided into those with an arteriovenous shunt and those without an arteriovenous shunt. With present diagnostic techniques, a genetic cause can be found in 10%–15% of cases.

* AVFs, nidal AVMs, and VGAMs are examples of vascular malformations with high-flow arteriovenous shunts.

* Cavernomas, DVAs, and Sturge–Weber syndrome are examples of intracranial vascular malformations without arteriovenous shunting.

* High-flow vascular malformations, particularly VGAMs, though rare, are an important cause of high-output cardiac failure and pulmonary hypertension. These clinical signs can be misinterpreted as a primary cardiac problem.

- A neonate presenting in heart failure secondary to a high-flow arteriovenous shunt is at high risk of significant morbidity and mortality.

- High-flow vascular malformations can present in childhood with macrocephaly, motor delay, papilloedema, and hydrocephalus due to venous hypertension.

- AVMs, although rare, are the most common cause of non-traumatic intracranial haemorrhage in childhood. Aneurysms are less common but can also present with intracranial haemorrhage.

- Careful clinical assessment and multimodality imaging, including CT, MRI, and cerebral angiography, followed by multidisciplinary discussion is essential for planning the management of intracranial vascular abnormalities.

- Although invasive, cerebral angiography is still the gold standard investigation for intracranial vascular anomalies with arteriovenous shunts.

- Treatment options include endovascular treatment with embolic agents, neurosurgical microsurgical resection, and stereotactic radiosurgery. Treatment is carried out in specialised neurovascular centres by skilled and experienced teams. Treatment choice requires multidisciplinary team discussion and appropriate counselling for patients and families.

- Careful follow-up without active intervention is a valid strategy for management of unruptured AVMs, but thresholds for treatment may be different from adults due to the lifelong risk of haemorrhage.

# REFERENCES

1. Duran D, Zeng X, Jin SC, Choi J, Nelson-Williams C, et al. Mutations in Chromatin modifier and ephrin signaling genes in vein of Galen malformation. *Neuron*. 2019 Feb 6;101(3):429–443.
2. Mohr JP, Parides MK, Stapf C, Moquete E, Moy CS, Overbey JR, Al-Shahi Salman R, Vicaut E, Young WL, Houdart E, Cordonnier C, Stefani MA, Hartmann A, von Kummer R, Biondi A, Berkefeld J, Klijn CJ, Harkness K, Libman R, Barreau X, Moskowitz AJ. International ARUBA investigators. Medical management with or without interventional therapy for unruptured brain arteriovenous malformations (ARUBA): A multicentre, non-blinded, randomised trial. *Lancet*. 2014 Feb 15;383(9917):614–621.
3. Gross BA, Storey A, Orbach DB, Scott RM, Smith ER. Microsurgical treatment of arteriovenous malformations in pediatric patients: The Boston Children's Hospital experience. *J Neurosurg Pediatr*. 2015 Jan;15(1):71–77.
4. Spetzler RF, Martin NA. A proposed grading system for arteriovenous malformations. *J Neurosurg*. 1986 Oct;65(4):476–483.
5. Lawton MT, Kim H, McCulloch CE, Mikhak B, Young WL. A supplementary grading scale for selecting patients with brain arteriovenous malformations for surgery. *Neurosurgery*. 2010 Apr;66(4):702–713.
6. Lauzier DC, Vellimana AK, Chatterjee AR, Osbun JW, Moran CJ, Zipfel GJ, Kansagra AP. Return of the lesion: A meta-analysis of 1134 angiographically cured pediatric arteriovenous malformations. *J Neurosurg Pediatr*. 2021 Sep 10;28(6):677–684. doi: 10.3171/2021.6.PEDS21227.
7. Bal J, Milosevich E, Rennie A, Robertson F, Toolis C, Bhate S, James G, Ganesan V. Management of haemorrhagic stroke secondary to arteriovenous malformations in childhood. *Childs Nerv Syst*. 2021 Apr;37(4):1255–1265.
8. Dinca EB, de Lacy P, Yianni J, Rowe J, Radatz MW, Preotiuc-Pietro D, Kemeny AA. Gamma knife surgery for pediatric arteriovenous malformations: A 25-year retrospective study. *J Neurosurg Pediatr*. 2012 Nov;10(5):445–450.
9. Cavernomas A Randomised Effectiveness (CARE) Study trial website: https://www.ed.ac.uk/usher/edinburgh-clinical-trials/our-studies/all-current-studies/care/care-study
10. Gross BA, Du R, Orbach DB, Scott RM, Smith ER, Bhate S, James G, Ganesan V. The natural history of cerebral cavernous malformations in children. *J Neurosurg Pediatr*. 2016 Feb;17(2):123–128.

# Index

index

index

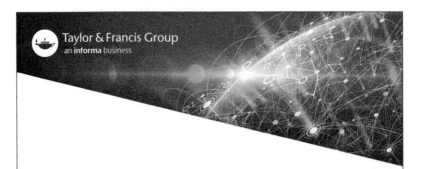

Printed and bound by CPI Group (UK) Ltd, Croydon, CR0 4YY

17/10/2024

01775698-0006